Top Tips for GPs

A beginner's guide to general practice

✗ Marking noted ocr'15 ✗·

Radcl

© 2000 Knut Schroeder

Radcliffe Medical Press Ltd
18 Marcham Road, Abingdon, Oxon OX14 1AA

British Library Cataloguing in Publication Data

A catalogue record for this book is available from the British Library.

ISBN 1 85775 440 9

Typeset by Joshua Associates Ltd, Oxford
Printed and bound by TJ International Ltd, Padstow, Cornwall

Contents

Foreword

This book is designed to guide the newcomer to the increasingly complex world of general practice, who may easily become bewildered by the wide variety of unfamiliar situations encountered and by the equally numerous pieces of good advice that are proffered from a variety of well-meaning sources. So often the appropriate advice does not arrive at the same time as the situation in which it would be most beneficial.

Knut Schroeder has put together, in a readily accessible form, those pieces of advice that he has found most helpful in his own experience as a registrar. He has brought an enthusiastic, observant and critical mind to bear on the everyday process of general practice. The author has canvassed widely, considered deeply and organised carefully to produce chapters which are not only informative but a pleasure to read either singly or as a continuum. While some chapters, such as those concerned with summative assessment and the MRCGP examination, are relevant mainly to the early years of practice, others could be perused with profit by the doctor further along in his or her career.

This is not a textbook of general practice but a distillation of many small pieces of wisdom, some of which may prove to have large benefits for those acting upon them. The ideas put forward will lead the new registrar along a path towards effective practice – and may indeed rehabilitate the more senior practitioner who wandered from such a path long ago.

The book brings together much information which is otherwise difficult to collate. It offers many ideas which should inspire examination of and experimentation with the way we work and the milieu in which we do so.

In short, it is strongly recommended for each new registrar and every training practice.

John Valentine
Course Organiser, Bath Vocational Training Scheme
Past Examiner, Royal College of General Practitioners
January 2000

Preface

This book aims to provide a few ideas to experiment with in the early stages of the registrar year, which has become busier in recent times. It is not meant to be either prescriptive or comprehensive, but rather it suggests ways to cope during the first few months and perhaps beyond. Some of these ideas may help you to create more time for your patients, your family and friends – and, of course, yourself.

Because general practice is complex, a short book like this cannot pretend to offer any easy solutions to what are often complicated questions. It certainly needs to be backed up both by reading the literature and by the training you will receive. There is always more than one way of doing things, and there is no guarantee that any of the ideas mentioned will work for you. However, if some of the suggestions help you to develop your own individual style, perhaps with completely different approaches, much will have been gained.

I would be extremely grateful to receive any comments or criticism regarding the contents of the book, or indeed some of your own 'hot tips'.

Don't panic! I hope you enjoy your registrar year!

Knut Schroeder
January 2000

Acknowledgements

I owe my greatest debts to two of my teachers, Chris Bevan and John Valentine, who by their inspiration and enthusiasm for general practice have greatly influenced my education. Without their generous support, kind encouragement and gentle advice this book would never have been written.

I would like to point out that most of the credit for the ideas in this book must go to all the general practitioners (especially Mark Dinwoodie, Jeremy Gilbert and Ruth Gillies at Fairfield Park Health Centre, Bath, and Michael Kirwin at the Mount Carmel Family Practice Center, Columbus, Ohio) and colleagues from other healthcare professions who so unselfishly passed on their experience and wisdom during my own training.

I should especially like to thank my friend and colleague Hazel Everett for her immensely useful comments and wonderful ideas.

The following GP colleagues from the Division of Primary Health Care at Bristol University have been most generous with their constructive criticisms and suggestions on earlier drafts of the manuscript: Tom Fahey, Anna Graham, Clare Grant, David Jewell, David Memel, Jo Protheroe, Chris Salisbury, Debbie Sharp, Nigel Stocks and Helen Stoddart. Through their contributions and my conversations with them I have learned so much more about general practice.

My wife Sharmila Choudhury has been a source of continuing support – and of subtle comments that led to a number of almost complete rewrites. Many thanks for opening my eyes to those numerous garbled sentences.

A big thank you of course to Nikki Dibley for kindly drawing the wonderful cartoons.

I am also very grateful to an anonymous reviewer who kindly

made many useful suggestions and drew my attention to the weak points in a previous draft.

Finally, I would like to express my gratitude to everyone at Radcliffe Medical Press, especially Heidi Allen, for their encouragement, moral support, help and enthusiasm, and for making this book possible.

Although I received a great deal of help from all concerned, I take sole responsibility for all opinions expressed and for any misinterpretations of others' ideas.

1 Finding your feet: starting as a registrar in general practice

Gencral practice is great fun – for most of the time. Working independently within the primary healthcare team and building relationships with all kinds of interesting people is very enjoyable. It can be absolutely fascinating to get to know your patients and to hear their sometimes incredible stories. A consultation that has gone well, where you and your patient managed to strike a similar chord, can be one of the most satisfying experiences. However, starting as a registrar in general practice may sometimes feel daunting, disorientating or even lonely. Many new registrars have worked in hospitals, often for a number of years, and are used to working in a team, sharing responsibility and treating serious conditions. However, beginning to make more decisions on your own and having only a few minutes rather than half an hour with a patient can be a little unsettling at first. And not knowing what to do (like everyone else starting as a registrar) when faced for the first time with common, simple problems such as head lice, ingrown toenails or emergency contraception may be frustrating and disheartening – but it does not have to be so. Hopefully the following pages contain some ideas that may help to make the transition from hospital medicine to primary care a little easier.

Looking for a training post

The decision to become a general practitioner can be made at various stages in one's medical career. Some doctors embark on their GP training straight after house jobs, whereas others try out a variety of hospital posts first. Registrars entering general practice may therefore have quite different backgrounds and skills. As individual practices vary widely, probably much more so than hospital posts, it is often worth shopping around to find a practice that suits you personally.

Choosing a type of vocational training

To become a fully qualified general practitioner you will need to work for two years in approved hospital posts and for one year as a registrar in general practice. There are different ways of obtaining the relevant experience, and one of them is to join a vocational training scheme. This usually comes as a package with a variety of hospital posts and a year in general practice, which is frequently split into two separate periods at the beginning and end of the training. One advantage of joining such a training scheme is that all your jobs will usually be in the same area, so you will not need to move house. In addition, you only have to apply once for the whole scheme, so it is not necessary to go for interviews every few months. However, flexibility may be limited, and you may be assigned a practice without choice. Those who already have considerable hospital experience may get some of their posts accredited for general practice training. However, it is possible to choose hospital posts and a registrar job individually, and to design your own scheme, but in those cases it is essential to confirm in advance with the Joint Committee on Postgraduate Training for General Practice or the Regional Adviser that all of the posts will be suitable for accreditation.

Applying for a vocational training scheme

Vacancies on GP training schemes are advertised in the job section of the *British Medical Journal* and the free GP press (available in most postgraduate libraries). However, if you are keen to work in a particular area, try to find out about a local scheme some time in advance. The postgraduate secretaries are usually extremely helpful and can provide information about both the scheme and the area. They may also be able to put you in contact with current senior house officers (SHOs) and registrars, who can be an invaluable source of information.

Preparing for the interview

All GP training schemes are different, and again the most useful advice about the format and contents of the interview can often be obtained from current registrars. Generally speaking, two of the questions you are likely to be asked concern your motivation to become a GP and the current hot topics in general practice – which are usually the ones that make some of the headlines in the free GP newspapers. Reading the latest editions spanning at least the preceding few months should give you a feel for important current issues, and you should try to form your own opinion on these topics.

Choosing a practice

Individual practices vary enormously, and it may be difficult to know what to look for when applying for a registrar post. It may help to think about whether you would like to work in a rural or urban practice in the future. If you want to see what a particular working area is like, choose a similar practice for your training, but if you are sure about your future plans, you may want to gain a different experience while you are training. Would you prefer a single-handed practice or a large surgery with an extensive primary healthcare team and many principals? Are you interested in complementary medicine or any other special features of a practice?

Selecting a trainer

When choosing a training practice, one of the most important aspects to consider is, of course, your prospective trainer. Trainers vary widely with regard to style and experience, and although they undergo regular training and assessment, fortunately they are individuals with different approaches to teaching and GP work in general. Would you prefer a younger or older trainer? Is their gender an important consideration? Are you keen that your future trainer has special interests that you may want to learn about, such as a special clinical area, police work or complementary medicine? What would your timetable look like, and how much protected time would you have for training? Again, it can be most useful to talk to one of the current or previous registrars about these issues.

Thinking general practice

Moving from hospital into primary care

General practice differs from hospital medicine in many ways. Acute minor illness and chronic disease are common medical presentations, and are sometimes woven into a complex psycho-logical or social background. Hospital medicine is often focused on treating disease, whereas in general practice it is much more often the individual who is the centre of attention and who happens to present with a particular condition. In addition, empirical treat-ment is much more common, and 'routine' investigations are mainly performed when they are clinically indicated. Investigations are also far less readily available, and it may take a number of days for a laboratory report to reach your in-tray after you have arranged an investigation. All of this can take a while to get used to when starting in general practice, but usually everything falls into place fairly quickly.

Learning about the 'practice culture'

All general practices have their own individual history and are staffed by different personalities. Over the years, most practices have developed their own way of working. Try to take your 'hospital hat' off when starting as a registrar, and use the first few weeks to get a feel of how your practice runs. How do team members communicate? Is there a hierarchy within the practice? What is the practice philosophy? Answers to these and similar questions can often only be found with time, so a period of careful observation may help you to find your place in the practice team. Finding out about the 'practice culture' is also important should you want to suggest any changes with regard to training or other issues that affect the practice organisation. Many 'odd' ways of working have their own history which justifies them, so try not to be too judgemental initially if you do not agree with a particular way of doing things.

Shaping your own education

Self-directed learning

As a registrar, you have the opportunity and privilege to take part in planning, shaping and organising your own training and education. Much of your learning will be based on your personal educational needs, so it is usually a good idea to perform a SWOT (strengths, weaknesses, opportunities and threats) analysis with your trainer, and to use this as a basis for planning the year ahead. This means putting all of the SWOT factors on paper, which will enable you and your trainer to keep your learning objectives in focus and to review your progress at a later stage. There are various ways in which you may learn about general practice, and you will play a large part in deciding on the details of your training. The first few weeks may also provide you with the opportunity and time to think about your longer-term career goals, and to attempt to incorporate certain aspects of training into your registrar year accordingly.

Getting the most out of tutorials

Tutorials are often held as one-to-one sessions with your trainer or another member of the primary healthcare team, and should take place in protected time. You may occasionally discover that some topics relevant to general practice may not have been covered adequately during your hospital jobs. Areas about which many registrars frequently feel ignorant or in which they lack confidence include ENT, dermatology, issuing certificates and family planning. These subjects can be tackled in various ways – for example, by arranging a tutorial with the most knowledgeable partner in the practice, or by attending hospital clinics or family planning sessions. In most cases your trainer will be able to help you find out what is relevant for your work in general practice. Good initial guides as to what is relevant include the trainer's report for summative assessment and lists of core knowledge and skills that can be obtained from your Regional Office for Summative Assessment. These can look quite overwhelming initially, but you won't need to know everything at once, so don't despair!

Selecting different ways of learning

People have different ideas about teaching and training, and to some extent you will be able to influence how, for example, your tutorials take place. You may opt to discuss difficult or unusual cases, talk about particular medical conditions, or perform a 'random case analysis', which means keeping the case-notes of one of your surgeries and discussing patients and your management at random. Another useful method of learning is to have joint appointments with your trainer or another partner, with both of you consulting in alternate sessions and discussing patients and aspects of the consultation. Acting out tricky consultations through role-play with your trainer is great fun and might give you more insight than you would ever expect. You may also want to use other resources outside the practice, such as attending GP sessions at the local shelter or family planning clinics.

Taking your time

Most GPs see patients at 5- to 10-minute intervals, depending on the practice and the type of appointment (i.e. routine or urgent). Many practices book registrar appointments at longer intervals initially, but you or your trainer may wish to move on very quickly to a shorter appointment time. However, it takes a little while to develop the ability to consult quickly, and you should probably try to resist the temptation to rush this, and negotiate with your trainer to keep longer appointments for as long as is necessary. To start with, 20-minute appointments usually give you plenty of time to get used to everything and to consult comfortably. You will also have enough time to nip out and ask your trainer or another team member any questions that may arise. Once you are more experienced, you can cut down the appointment time to 15 minutes and later to 10 minutes or shorter. You will benefit for your whole GP career if you try to take your time initially and aim to learn things properly. It is a little like learning how to play a musical instrument – only slow and controlled practice at the beginning will enable you to become fluent and fast later. However slowly you start, try to work towards having the same caseload and appointment length as the other partners in the practice at the end of the year, or preferably a little earlier. In this way you will get used to the average GP workload, which can make locum work or starting as a new principal much easier.

Setting your timetable

Usually you will discuss your timetable early on with your trainer or the practice manager. This is not written in stone, and normally there is room for debate. As registrars come from different back-grounds, their experience and confidence vary. Some may be quite happy to work almost by themselves after a fairly brief introductory period, while others may need much more time before they are able to work more independently. Try not to be pressurised into working patterns with which you do not feel comfortable, and if necessary even revert to longer appointments or more supervision if you find that a change took place too quickly. You will almost certainly be very busy after a few months, so enjoy the first few weeks and use the time to get to know everything and everyone in the practice.

Getting to know your team

Finding out about your colleagues in the practice

The first few weeks are the best time to learn the names of all the members of the primary healthcare team and to get to know everyone personally. All of the patients on the practice list are usually looked after together by the whole primary healthcare team, with more or less input from different team members. Once you have started, use every opportunity to visit and meet your working colleagues, including receptionists, practice and community nurses, health visitor, community midwife, secretaries and practice man-ager. There may also be others attached to your practice, such as a counsellor, psychologist, physiotherapist or chiropodist. They don't usually bite, and will generally be very keen to meet you if you show an interest in what they are doing. Introduce yourself and find out how you can contact them and how they would contact you (e.g. via communication books, messages, regular meetings, etc.). Learn about their roles and working patterns, and ask if you can sit in with any of them at some stage. You will be amazed how much you can learn, for example, from the practice nurse (about chronic disease management, dealing with small injuries, dressings, etc.), the health visitor (about child health surveillance, etc.), the occupational therapist/physiotherapist (about use of aids for daily living, rehabilitation, etc.) or the practice manager (about practice finance, practice management, etc.). This will not only deepen your understanding of their roles and how the practice runs, but is commonly excellent preparation for summative assessment and the MRCGP, as you may learn many things that are difficult to extract from textbooks.

Learning about other services in the community

Once you have got to know everyone in the practice, you should make a great effort to find out about other community services in your area. I cannot overemphasise how useful it is to know what support is available outside your practice. Important members of the primary healthcare team and other resources include, for example, social services, the local hospice and palliative care team, community occupational therapists, incontinence advisers, specialist nurses (e.g. diabetic, health promotion, cardiology, etc.), a variety of counselling services (e.g. in relation to drugs, alcohol, psychiatric disorders, gambling, marital problems, etc.), patient self-help groups and many others. The registrar year, with ample opportunity for training, is the ideal time to get to know the roles and availability of all of these services, and this will be extremely beneficial both for your patients and for your own support.

Designing the consulting room

Obtain the basic equipment

Surgeries vary with regard to the standard and equipment of their consulting rooms. Most training practices will provide you with your own consulting room, but you may sometimes find that you have to share a room with another colleague. Aim to collect all of the necessary equipment for your room if it is not fully stocked.

Try to avoid running out of equipment, as it can be very frustrating if you have to interrupt a surgery in order to obtain blood bottles or swabs because there are none left. Find out at an early stage who is responsible for replacing consumables (in most cases it will probably be you, but in some practices this is done by the receptionist or the practice nurse), so that you know who to

---

Table 1.1 Consulting-room equipment

1 Stationery
- Prescription pad
- Medical certificates
- Laboratory forms (haematology, biochemistry, immunology, microbiology)
- X-ray/ultrasound/other imaging forms
- Referral forms (chiropody, occupational therapy, physiotherapy, counselling, palliative care, etc.)
- Patient continuation cards (male and female)
- Headed notepaper and envelopes
- Dictation equipment (machine and empty tapes)
- Patient information leaflets
- Spare pens

2 Reference
- *British National Formulary*
- *Oxford Handbook of Clinical Medicine*
- *Oxford Handbook of Clinical Specialties*
- Practice formulary and local clinical guidelines
- Chief Medical Officer's communications
- Local laboratory handbook
- Contact details of primary healthcare team (GPs, practice nurse, receptionist, midwife, community nurse, physiotherapist, palliative care team)
- Telephone directory

- Local maps
- Height/weight conversion charts
- Fitness-to-drive leaflet

3 Examination
- Ophthalmoscope/auriscope/torch with blue filter
- Spare earpieces
- Spare batteries
- Sphygmomanometer
- Tongue depressors
- Magnifying glass
- Tape measure
- Peak-flow meter with mouthpieces
- Fluorescein
- Snellen chart
- Examination gloves, lubricating jelly, tissues
- Specula (assorted)
- Examination couch
- Examination light
- Teddy for children/other toys/ stickers

4 Investigation
- Tourniquet, alcoholic wipes, needles, butterflies, cotton wool, plasters, syringes
- Blood bottles: haematology (FBC, clotting, group and save), biochemistry, immunology
- Pathology pots: urine, cytology, stool
- Microbiology: urine, blood culture, wound swabs, high vaginal swabs, chlamydia
- Urinalysis, glucose stix
- Box for used instruments
- Sharps box

contact if your supplies run low. To make it easier for yourself or the person replenishing these items, write a list of the things you like to have in stock and put it up close to your clinical area (e.g. on the wall or inside the cupboard door). This will serve as a reminder and make it much easier to identify what has or is about to run out.

Start afresh and clear out any unnecessary items

We all have different needs and requirements, so it may be an idea to think of furniture or equipment that you require for consulting, examining, performing procedures, administration or video-taping. If important items of equipment are missing, ask whether there are any in the practice, and if not whether they could be ordered. Get rid of any clutter or outdated items that might have accumulated over the years. Find the best location for your furniture, where it both 'feels right' and is practical. You also need to think about personal security when arranging your room, and it is important to keep your exits clear in case you have to deal with an aggressive patient. Make sure that your consulting room is patient-friendly and allows easy access for the elderly, parents with children and disabled patients.

Find the most appropriate room layout for your personal style

You will spend a large proportion of your time in your consulting room, so it is important to make it comfortable and suitable for your daily work. Most consulting rooms are well-equipped for routine surgeries, but you will find that you may have very personal requirements with regard to desk position, equipment and internal decoration. Individual styles with regard to interior design vary tremendously, and a little of the 'Changing Rooms' approach may help to make your room more comfortable and friendly. A few of your favourite pictures and a couple of plants can make quite a difference. Some GPs display photographs of their family, children's drawings or some object that reflects their personal interests. This often attracts attention and can break the ice with difficult patients, as well as providing a more relaxing environment in which to work.

Customise your clinical area

It is likely that you will need to perform various clinical procedures in your consulting room. Adequate lighting is important, and is absolutely essential for certain examinations. It is good practice to have separate workplaces for clean and dirty procedures, and to keep all of the frequently required items laid out in an orderly manner on a worktop, tray or trolley where they are easily accessible. Have a lined bin at close range and a sharps box nearby, but out of reach of children.

Place health information material next to the patient's chair

It is easy to position a small shelf close to the patient's chair with information leaflets on contraception, health promotion, etc. This can encourage curiosity, and patients often pick up and read leaflets if you have to leave the room, prepare for a procedure, telephone the hospital or fill out a form. It is amazing how often this stimulates questions such as 'I didn't know you could get emergency contraception' or 'I often wanted to stop smoking but never knew that there are things that can help me', resulting in more awareness of available services or treatments.

File patient information leaflets

Most practices keep a supply of (often excellent) patient information leaflets. Some of them can be very helpful for backing up topics that you may discuss with the patient during the consultation, and patients can take them home to read at leisure. A filing cabinet or drawer containing useful leaflets, ordered from A to Z according to specific conditions, is often a good system for storage, and allows quick retrieval. In addition, many visual aids and items such as placebo inhalers or a collection of contraceptive devices can make explanation and demonstration to patients easier.

Provide extra seats for individuals accompanying the patient

Many patients bring relatives or friends along with them, so it can be useful to have at least one extra chair available. If you do not have enough space in your room, a couple of spare chairs can usually be placed in the corridor outside your room where they are readily accessible.

Keep a toy box for children

Patients frequently bring their children along to the consultation, which is usually very pleasant and can brighten up your session. However, small children tend to get bored very quickly and may soon start investigating your room and equipment, unless you have something more interesting prepared for them, such as a toy box. If you do not have children of your own, ask some of your colleagues or other young parents which toys are currently in vogue, as many apparently interesting ones only occupy attention for a few seconds! In this way you may also be able to gather a few 'donations' of unused or unwanted items. Try to choose quiet toys that will make listening through your stethoscope or talking to the parent less of a struggle. Collect a few larger toys rather than too many small ones, as undoubtedly you will be the one who has to clear up before the next patient comes in! Toys can also be useful aids when examining children (*see also* Chapter 2 on effective consultations).

Locate the emergency buzzer

It is useful to know whether your room has an emergency button that you can press if any situation gets out of control. You will probably rarely if ever need it, but you should know where it is located. Find out whether it works and who responds to it. You may also want to know how to switch the alarm off yourself in case you (or one of your patients) set it off accidentally.

Arranging your desk

Store all your most frequently needed articles of equipment in or around your desk

It can be very disruptive and time-wasting if you have keep having to get up from your chair during the consultation. Although being disorganised and having a cluttered desk can have its attractions, and you may personally favour this arrangement, on hectic days it often contributes to raising your stress levels. If you hate having to search for things, organise your desk and try to have all the regularly needed items ready to hand. For example, diagnostic aids and equipment for daily use can be stored together in a single drawer or in a small basket on your desktop. A small stock of empty recording tapes in your drawer will help to reduce delays when you want to dictate a letter. It is also a good idea to move your computer printer close by – if necessary on to a small table next to you – so that you can tear off newly printed prescriptions easily without having to get up from your chair. Make sure that you have a lockable drawer or cupboard for storing your prescription pad and other valuable or confidential items.

Write a list of all essential telephone numbers

Most practices have a directory of important telephone numbers. If not, consult the phone book and compile your own list. In addition, you could phone a secretary in the general hospital office and ask whether she could send you an internal hospital directory. This will be of great value if you want to phone the laboratory or some other hospital department directly without going through the hospital switchboard.

Table 1.2 Important telephone numbers

- Ambulance control (acute admissions and outpatients)
- Casualty
- Chemists
- Community nurses
- Co-operative/deputising service
- Coroner's Office
- Delivery suite
- Eye clinic
- Family planning clinic
- Genito-urinary clinic
- Health authority
- Home care
- Hospital Results Service
- Local hospitals/bed bureaus
- Local self-help groups
- Mental health team
- Miscarriage Association
- Palliative care service
- Poison information centres
- Police
- Practice: partners (also home/ mobile numbers)
- Public health (notifiable disease)
- Reception
- Social services
- Special care baby unit
- Undertaker

Find out how to refer

Ask your practice whether any local referral guidelines exist, and note down how and where to refer for the commonest problems. The practice may also have special referral forms. You could ask all of the partners in the practice to routinely arrange a photocopy of letters from local hospitals outlining new procedures, local guidelines or protocols, and to put them in a special file for locums and registrars. It is also worth having a tutorial on whom to refer to for particular conditions, as some consultants may have a special interest in certain areas.

Have the most important references in front of you

It is impossible to have every piece of information that you need for everyday general practice at your fingertips – and this is not expected of you. For this reason, keep the most commonly used reference books, such as the *British National Formulary*, an emergency folder with the latest protocols, clinical references, a notebook with important addresses and telephone numbers, practice guidelines and your diary on your desk. In addition, you can store height/weight and conversion charts and anatomical diagrams (to illustrate points to your patient) in a clear plastic folder. Generally speaking, there is no need to be shy about looking things up in front of your patients. They often appreciate that you cannot know everything and are usually very pleased to see that you are checking up drug doses, for example, as a safeguard for their own benefit.

Write essential information on index cards

It is often difficult to find and remember facts such as the types of tests that need to be arranged prior to some referrals, or the required frequency of blood tests when titrating drug doses, especially if you need such information quickly. To make access to this type of information easier, it can be helpful to have on your desk a small filing box of alphabetically ordered topics written on index cards containing all those relevant facts that may be difficult to locate and are easy to forget. It only takes a few seconds to note down hot tips from your trainer, or recommendations from the hospital consultant, or to cut out and glue down useful lists from the GP journals, quickly adding to your personal collection of general practice-specific knowledge. If your practice is fully computerised, you could record this information using a word-processing package or a spreadsheet program.

Shed light on the confusing array of stationery

The variety of forms and paperwork that are needed can be a little disorientating for beginners in general practice. As it is relatively important to know your way round sick notes and medical reports, try to devote a tutorial with your trainer to this topic quite early on. Find out which forms are most frequently needed, and keep a constant supply of them available. If you have a practice stamp, try to have as many forms as possible pre-stamped, which will save you having to fill out practice details by hand.

Try to minimise body tension

Having a comfortable chair will help you to survive and even enjoy long surgeries, as sitting in an awkward position can lead to tension and discomfort. Your chair and desk need to be at the correct height to support your posture, and if necessary you can easily raise the desk slightly by putting small pieces of wooden board under the legs. This often makes a dramatic difference, especially if you are tall. Try to obtain a comfortable chair if you do not already have one – your practice may be very accommodating in this respect.

Find the right place for your computer screen

Having to turn away frequently during your consultation can be disruptive and may result in your missing occasional important patient cues. For this reason, placing your computer screen in your line of sight when facing your patient can be helpful, as you will then be able to maintain eye contact for most of the time. You can still show your patients details on the screen by simply turning it around when required. However, some GPs would disagree with this, and prefer to place the screen at an angle of 90 degrees to the patient so that they can look at either the patient or the computer screen, so you may want to try out different options.

Learn to use the computer

Many practices provide a user's guide for new registrars or locums, and it is worth reading this and familiarising yourself with the computer if you do not want to struggle with it too much in front of patients. A variety of software packages is available with different advantages and drawbacks. If you are new to computers or to the medical software, try to obtain some basic training from your trainer or someone else in the practice who can show you the 'ins and outs'. Find out how to start and shut down the program used by the practice, and whether you need your own personal password. It is also essential to know how to book appointments, get the patient's records on to the screen and look at the drug history. It is important to learn as soon as possible how to process and alter acute and repeat prescriptions correctly. Practise entering various types of clinical and non-clinical information, and find out how to record payments for Item of Service. Remember that if it all seems too complicated at the beginning, you can be reassured that everyone else feels the same – but usually not for very long.

Use word-processing packages

Many practice computers have word-processing packages which can make your life much easier. It usually does not take very long to find your way round the commonly used software (although admittedly there is a learning curve). This will help you to produce high-quality reports (e.g. for your audit project), summaries for your study group and professional-looking CVs. If you have the time and inclination, it can also be very useful to learn touch-typing, as this can speed up your consultations and preparation of documents. However, it has to be said that it takes a little practice to become fluent in typing, and many people can achieve a tremendous speed even with two fingers!

The doctor's bag

Stock your doctor's bag

Training practices usually supply their registrar with a doctor's bag, but the amount and quality of the contents tend to vary. After the registrar year you will need your own bag, and you may decide to start collecting your own equipment sooner rather than later. However, bags and diagnostic tools are costly, and before you start to spend any money it is a good idea to ask your colleagues about their experiences with various articles of equipment or particular types of bags. If you regularly work in socially deprived areas and for personal safety reasons would prefer not to be immediately recognised as a doctor, you may want to consider using a rucksack or other casual bag instead. Whatever type of bag you buy, make sure that you can lock it.

Make a list of articles you need

With the help of your trainer, devise your own personal list of items which you can use to stock your bag. This is often a good topic for one of the first tutorials, when you can discuss management of emergencies and the use of drugs in general practice at the same time. It is tempting to accept free starter packs from pharmaceutical companies, but be aware that they often contain new drugs and more expensive ones than the medication you would normally prescribe. Moreover, they are not necessarily the most appropriate option for your patient.

Table 1.3 Suggested contents of the doctor's bag

1 Stationery
- GMS3 temporary services registration form
- Prescription pad/private prescriptions
- MED3 and MED5 forms
- X-ray and laboratory forms
- Practice's headed notepaper
- Pre-printed admission sheets (if available)
- Envelopes
- 'Post-it' notes
- Continuation cards (male/female), unless paperless
- Notebooks (bag refill, patient contacts, things to look up)
- Spare pens
- Dictating machine

2 Diagnostic equipment
- Thermometer
- Sphygmomanometer
- Stethoscope
- Electronic thermometer
- Auriscope/ophthalmoscope
- Fluorescein
- Torch
- Tendon hammer
- Peak-flow meter
- Glucostix + sterets, lancets, cotton wool and plasters
- Urine multistix
- Examination gloves, lubricating jelly, tissues
- Venepuncture set

3 References
- List of essential telephone numbers
- *British National Formulary* (BNF)
- *Oxford Handbook of Clinical Medicine*
- *Oxford Handbook of Clinical Specialties*
- Emergency cards
- Obstetric calendar
- Local maps

Table 1.4 Suggested selection of drugs for the doctor's bag (NB: Please check with your trainer and local guidelines)

- Analgesia (assorted drugs, including paracetamol, NSAIDs)
- Anti-emetic
- Antibiotics (penicillin, non-penicillin alternatives, eye ointment)
- Antihistamine
- Cardiac: diamorphine (+ naloxone), aspirin, glyceryl trinitrate (GTN) spray, atropine, diuretic, adrenaline
- Asthma: hydrocortisone, salbutamol
- Fits: rectal diazepam
- Hypoglycaemia: glucose, glucagon
- Renal colic: pethidine or diclofenac
- Syntometrine

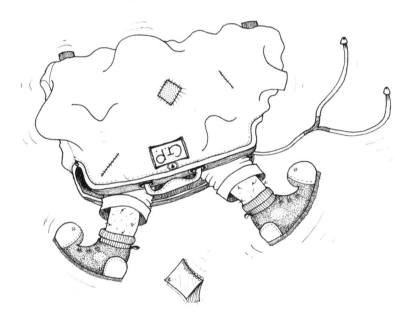

Keep your drugs and other items up to date

Some GPs carry a small notebook in their bag for jotting down items that have started to run low and need to be replaced. Find out where drugs and other equipment are kept in the surgery, so that you know where to obtain new supplies. In general, it is probably best to keep the amount and number of drugs as low as possible and to restock rather more frequently. Check the contents of your bag regularly (e.g. every one to two months) to ensure that they have not exceeded their expiry date. If you obtain your drugs from a chemist, ensure that all the packs have their expiry date and batch number clearly visible. This is for your own protection as much as for patients' safety, as you may, after a couple of months or even longer, need to trace where a drug has come from if there has been an unsuspected complication due to a drug reaction. It is your responsibility to keep your prescriptions and controlled drugs locked away both in your surgery and at home. The introductory pages of the *British National Formulary* (BNF) provide useful guidance on this and other prescribing issues.

Keep rarely used items in a separate bag

It is very tempting to try to cater for all eventualities, but your bag would become so heavy that you would not be able to carry it five yards! For this reason it might be helpful to decide which articles of equipment you think you always need to carry with you. Keep only small numbers of items such as blood bottles and syringes in your main bag, and store spares or infrequently used gadgets and pots in separate bags that you can keep in your car. Prepare emergency packs for your bag in the manner described later in this chapter, as these are particularly useful in small or dark homes where treating emergencies and finding all of the required bits and pieces can sometimes be rather a challenge.

Table 1.5 Suggested items for an additional bag

- Specimen bottles (urine plain and boric acid, stool)
- Swabs (wound/high vaginal/ chlamydia)
- Venepuncture spares (needles, bottles, alcoholic wipes, cotton wool, plasters, specimen bags)
- Dressing pack
- Syringes (assorted)
- Needles (assorted)
- Sterile gloves
- Sharps box
- Single-use speculum
- Venflons and butterflies (assorted)
- Infusion set
- Haemaccel
- Saline (0.9%) for infusion
- Laerdal pocket mask, oropharyngeal airways
- Water for injection
- Saline flush (0.9%)
- Nebuliser

Using your car

Keep your car in good working order

A reliable car is essential, especially in rural areas where home visits can involve many miles of driving. It is essential to be able to get to emergencies promptly, so your car will need to be in good condition. You do not need to drive the latest model, and an old car can be just as dependable, but investing in a car service and getting any necessary repairs completed before you take up your post is often money well spent.

Get ready for winter night visits

Cold weather can make visiting fairly unpleasant unless you are prepared for chilly conditions. If you work in hilly countryside, make sure that your tyres are in good condition, and keep some warm clothes in the car in case you break down. In the event of a flat battery, a pair of jump leads can be very useful, and they are relatively inexpensive. Cold steering wheels can make subsequent examination of a patient difficult, and using warm gloves when you are in your car or outside during a chilly winter will be much kinder to both the patient and yourself.

Obtain all of the essential basic clinical equipment for your car

One important difference between seeing patients in their homes and at the surgery is that you have to take everything that you need with you on a home visit. Running out of supplies in your consulting room is not normally a major problem, as spares are usually easy to obtain. However, not having your prescription pad, spare blood bottles or a nebuliser with you can make life very difficult if you are on a visit far away from your practice. Therefore it is important to keep your car and your bags well equipped with all the clinical and stationery items that you regularly need.

Working out of hours

Check your equipment before going on duty

It can sometimes be rather difficult to obtain spare drugs or equipment in the middle of the night. Make sure that your drug supply and emergency equipment are up to date and in working order. If you are on call for a co-operative, it is helpful to find out which drugs and equipment are available to you and whether they are in stock in sufficient quantity. Check that essential items such as the nebuliser are working properly. You may also want to write down and keep the telephone number of a back-up GP in case the situation suddenly becomes very serious (this will usually be your trainer or another partner during the registrar year).

Keep separate records for yourself

Co-operatives and deputising firms normally send faxes or copies of consultation notes out of hours directly to the patient's practice. Particularly in difficult or delicate cases, it is worth keeping your own records in a small notebook just in case there are any problems later on. Many GPs also write down the batch number and expiry date of every drug they supply while on duty, which does require a little time and effort, but may be important at a later stage for medico-legal reasons.

Ask your patient to help you to find the right house in the dark

In some areas, locating your patient's home can be time-consuming. Cars are sometimes much more distinctive than houses, so you could ask your patient to tell you the type of car parked in front of the house, together with the number-plate details. Switching on the hazard lights of the car would make it even more obvious and recognisable. You could also ask for all the lights in the house to be left on. It is essential to take your patient's telephone number and carry it with you in case you have difficulty in finding the right house and need to obtain further directions. A strong torch (you could buy one that is powered by the car cigarette lighter) can be useful if street signs or house numbers are difficult to see. Obtain a detailed street map of your practice area and, if necessary, road plans of local housing estates in case streets are not signposted.

Making contact

Before you do your first practice on-call or out-of-hours shift on your own (which is normally not for some time), it is essential that you know how the communication links between practice and duty doctor work. Most practices use either mobile phones or pagers, which can occasionally be a little confusing to use if you are unfamiliar with them, so try to talk through the procedures and discuss the necessary equipment with your trainer. It is important to find out whether there are any problem zones within your practice area where your mobile phone may have a poor connection. Make an effort to let the receptionists know if you are leaving the practice premises and when you expect to be back. This may save you being contacted about a relatively non-urgent problem that could have waited until your return to the surgery.

General practice emergencies

Prepare yourself for emergencies

Most practices have an induction period of variable length, with registrars mainly sitting in with their trainer or other partners to begin with, but relatively soon you will start seeing patients on your own. Don't panic. Emergencies occur relatively rarely in general practice, but they do nevertheless happen from time to time. It is fairly unlikely that you will face any major life-threatening conditions within the first few days. However, even a condition that you will encounter on average only once a year might challenge you during your first consultation. For this reason, try to get prepared for treating emergencies both in and out of the surgery as soon as you start seeing patients on your own.

Know where to find the necessary equipment

You will probably need to find out fairly soon where drugs and other emergency equipment such as nebulisers or a defibrillator (if available) are located in your surgery, and how to obtain help quickly (e.g. via an intercom system or panic button). Ask for a brief introduction to the way in which the emergency equipment works, and refresh your knowledge regularly. Your surgery may also have its own policy with regard to various emergency treatments. This is worth knowing about, as the arrangements for treating emergencies can vary widely depending on both practice area and access to secondary services.

Note down important telephone numbers

It can be very useful to keep a separate card or notebook containing important telephone numbers, especially those that you may require in emergencies. This should include numbers for the hospital switchboard, ambulance control, social worker and any other services that you may need to contact urgently, especially out of hours. Also obtain the home and mobile telephone numbers of your colleagues in case you need to ask for advice or help from the partner who covers you. A good place to put a card or sticker listing useful telephone numbers is the inside of your bag – as the numbers will be immediately visible when you open it.

Have the necessary references to hand

Treating acute illness in general practice differs in many ways from the hospital setting. As emergency protocols for most conditions will be new to you, you may find it very helpful to collect the latest guidelines and recommendations from your trainer, and to keep copies of these in your consulting room and doctor's bag, preferably in a file.

Write out emergency cards for common and important emergencies

Guidelines and protocols can be difficult to use in an emergency situation, due to their size and layout. You may complement these by writing your own personal emergency summaries on index cards. Include only the essential information needed for diagnosis and treatment (e.g. drug doses and management steps) and order them alphabetically, and you will be able to use them as a quick reminder within seconds. Store them in your bag (e.g. near your emergency drugs) and on your desk, where they will often be invaluable should your mind go blank in a stressful situation. You will be able to update them or highlight certain changes quite easily, which is useful, as protocols and guidelines tend to change fairly frequently.

Prepare special bags for treating emergencies

When faced with an unexpected urgent situation, it can be difficult to locate all of the items you need for quick treatment. Although this happens very rarely, preparing your own condition-specific 'emergency packs' for your consulting room and your doctor's bag can be very useful. The packs should contain all of the important items of equipment that are needed for the most urgent scenarios, where it is important not to waste time searching for odd items that you need in a hurry. For example, a 'meningococcal septicaemia pack' could contain the following items: a small, clear plastic plate to check for a non-blanching rash, syringes, needles, the appropriate antibiotics with vials of water, a card with drug doses for children and adults, alcoholic wipes, blood culture bottles, a pair of gloves and whatever else you think you may need. All of this should fit into a small, clear plastic bag that you can label with the name of the condition as well as the expiry date of the medication. Bags can be prepared in a similar manner for other conditions (e.g. myocardial infarction or anaphylactic shock), enabling you to perform emergency treatments much more smoothly.

Making the most of the registrar year

Further postgraduate qualifications

Various diplomas, mainly oriented towards GPs, are available from some of the Royal Colleges. These include: the Diploma in Child Health (DCH) and the Diploma in Geriatric Medicine (DGM), both from the Royal College of Physicians; the Diploma in Obstetrics and Gynaecology (DRCOG) from the Royal College of Obstetricians and Gynaecologists; and the Diploma in Family Planning from the Faculty of Family Planning and Reproductive Health Care. Studying for these diplomas will certainly be useful for your work as a GP, can be a source of professional and personal satisfaction, and looks good on your CV. However, preparation for these qualifications needs to be taken seriously and requires considerable time and effort, and occasionally GP principals may feel threatened if you apply for a post in their practice and have a large collection of diplomas. The examination and course fees are also substantial and can eat significantly into your budget. If at all possible, try to sit the examinations during your hospital posts if you want to obtain any of these diplomas, as time will be at a premium during your registrar year and you may already have enough on your plate. Details about the format and requirements for the diplomas are available from the Royal Colleges, and often include SHO experience in that particular subject as well as passing written, clinical and oral examinations.

Signing up for health authority lists

For practices to receive payment for particular services, you often need to be included on special health authority lists. These include lists in obstetrics, child health surveillance and minor surgery. Different health authorities have varying inclusion requirements, and it is worth enquiring about these early on. In order to be admitted to the obstetric list you often need to have completed an SHO post in obstetrics and gynaecology and need evidence of experience in antenatal care and in attending normal and abnormal deliveries. There are national guidelines for child health surveillance, and a certificate of competence in performing child health surveillance is usually required. For the minor surgery list, experience in accident and emergency or other surgical skills (e.g. house jobs, minor surgery course) is necessary in most cases. Often you will need testimonials and signatures from the respective hospital consultants and, in general, having obtained the relevant diplomas will greatly enhance your eligibility. Admission to these lists will certainly be a bonus when you are applying for general practice posts later on.

Developing other interests

If you would like to develop other interests after or during the registrar year, it is often best to find out about this at an early stage. Research opportunities for GPs are improving, and many academic general practice departments will be keen to discuss with you any job prospects (*see also* Chapter 7 on career options). Many general practices teach medical students, and if you would like to obtain teaching experience this may also be a good time to get involved.

Looking at your contract

At the beginning of your registrar post you should have been given a work contract and asked to return a signed copy to the practice. Contracts may vary slightly from one practice to another, so it is important to read them thoroughly and discuss with your trainer or practice manager any areas about which you are not entirely happy. In particular, working hours, on-call commitments and other potentially delicate topics are much easier to sort out early on in your training year. Of course, the financial aspects have to be considered as well, and many of us are very hesitant about discussing such matters, but there a number of payments to which you are entitled. For example, the fees for your medical defence organisation will be reimbursed and you will receive a car allowance. Your vocational training scheme (VTS) may also pay certain travel expenses or course fees, and it is worth enquiring about this.

Thinking about personal financial protection

During the first few weeks you will undoubtedly be very busy settling into your new job. However, once the initial dust has settled, the beginning of the registrar year may be a good time to start sorting out matters such as your pension, critical illness cover and life insurance. Although this may sound a little boring, these arrangements could potentially be very important in the event of your falling ill, especially if you have a family and/or have taken on a mortgage. For example, the NHS pension scheme only pays for a certain length of time in the event of sudden inability to work due to illness. In order to make an informed decision about this, it is essential to obtain advice from an independent financial adviser. Financial advice is often offered free of charge (for instance by BMA financial services), and friends and GP colleagues will often be able to recommend a financial adviser to you.

2 Next please: aiming for effective consultations

Difficult or unpopular patients
Aggressive patients
Puzzling medical problems
Children
Adolescents
Record-keeping
Follow-up
Difficult home visits

Difficult or unpopular patients

The consultation is the central element of general practice, and becoming experienced in consultation skills may require many years of training and practice. However, one has to start somewhere. A short book like this cannot and does not intend even to outline the basics of consultation technique, and learning how to consult is part of the day-release course and training in your practice, backed up by reading the standard literature. Rather, this chapter aims to provide some simple suggestions (that may not always work!) on how to tackle some difficult or more unusual patient contacts that may be baffling when you are first starting work as a registrar. Generally speaking, the great majority of patients are undoubtedly very pleasant and enjoyable to look after. However, most general practitioners will invariably have a couple of characters among their patients who may cause an immediate 'fight-or-flight' reaction as soon as their name is spotted. These few people, who may have difficult personalities, exuberant demands or a multitude of problems, sometimes pose a definite challenge, making us doubt our own competence because we find it difficult to cater for their needs. A few strategies may help you to make the most of these encounters, resulting in a satisfactory consultation for both patient and doctor.

Try not to retreat from unpleasant patients

Almost all practices have some patients who may be unpleasant, dirty or smelly, or who display somewhat irritating behaviour. It is often all too easy to react in a judgemental way and to deny those patients the interest and attention that they deserve. Make it a habit to find out why and for how long a patient has been in a poor condition or has shown personal neglect. This approach often yields surprising results. A little detective work can be very rewarding, will increase your interest in the patient and may lead you to find a remediable reason for a particular presentation or behaviour. Flicking through the past history in the case-notes may also reveal a variety of more serious incidents that your patient may have experienced and which may be responsible for them being difficult or unusual. These experiences are sometimes of a more serious nature, and may include rape or physical or sexual abuse in the past, jail sentences, torture, kidnapping, accidents, a child's death or various other kinds of trauma that might not immediately cross your mind. You may never find an obvious cause, but knowing about a person's background may make you regard your patient with more empathy and therefore in a slightly different light.

Challenge your own attitudes

From time to time it is not the patient who is the main problem, but rather our own attitudes. It can be quite difficult to cope with failure, especially when our expectations are very high. You may be faced with a mountain of problems in a single patient, all of which are almost impossible to solve. In such cases it is sometimes helpful to sit back for a while and to try to form a realistic view of how much you and your patient may be able to achieve. Rather than expecting complete success in every patient with a chronic condition such as diabetes, hypertension or alcoholism, setting goals that are tailored to your patient is often far more practicable and worthwhile in the long term.

Value your achievements

Some patients can indeed be very hard work. You may struggle for months to resolve a medical or social problem, only to find at the end that your advice is being largely ignored. However, very often your input will have made some positive difference to your patient or the family involved, so it is often far better to concentrate on your successes, however small they may be, rather than on all those high expectations that you wanted to fulfil but never did.

Probe below the surface

If your patient presents with unusual symptoms, you may want to make it a priority to <u>find out what really lies behind</u> the complaints. From time to time, <u>vague symptoms</u> such as aches and pains indicate a deeper problem of a social, psychological, financial or sexual nature. Investing some initial time and effort in listening to and exploring the reasons for making an appointment, rather than quickly prescribing symptomatic relief, can save a considerable amount of time and fruitless effort in the long term. The simple question 'What do you think is wrong with you?' can sometimes produce surprising revelations about what is going on in your patient's mind.

Examine your patient

<u>Physical examination</u> is traditionally being taught as mainly <u>diagnostic</u>, but it can <u>also</u> be a very powerful <u>therapeutic</u> tool. Due to time constraints in general practice you will learn to focus your examination on the presenting problem, and at times it may become very tempting to take short cuts. However, even if you are sure from the history that a condition is benign, you can sometimes

only reassure your patient adequately if you examine the affected part of the body thoroughly. For instance, taking some time to explain that you are checking for signs of 'pressure in the head' when examining the cranial nerves in a patient with headache may be very helpful if there is an underlying concern about a brain tumour. Similarly, listening to a patient's chest could make a small but significant difference, as it may alleviate unfounded fears about a serious condition such as tuberculosis or cancer. Appropriate and thorough physical examination may reduce the number of follow-up consultations for reassurance if you can confidently lessen your patient's concerns and worries. On the other hand, you may sometimes uncover surprising findings that you would never have expected from the history. For many patients there is still some 'magic' in medicine, and using gadgets such as your ophthalmoscope may be a surprisingly effective form of treatment.

Break down patients' problem lists and tackle each problem individually

A small number of patients occasionally bring a long list of complaints with them into the consultation, and these are usually impossible to deal with in a single session. Take a deep breath and relax, as you do not need to solve all of the problems at once! Asking your patient to run through the whole list at the beginning can help to identify and prioritise the most important items. It is often much easier to come to an agreement when the boundaries and time constraints during a single consultation are made clear from the start. Most patients are happy if you prioritise their problems, so long as you indicate that you will attend to the rest of them at some stage.

Deflate patients' expectations

Influenced by reports in the media, some patients think that modern medicine is able to solve almost any medical problem. You will encounter individuals whose demands may be quite unreasonable with regard to their management, and this is often not their own fault but due to the incorrect or inadequate information that they have received. Rather than blaming patients for these high expectations, it is often more important to educate them and to make it clear that you are not omnipotent. For example, by saying 'It is highly unlikely that I'll be able to help in this matter, but I'll try' and explaining the reasons for your views, you may prepare the ground for a more rational discussion.

Demands for certificates

Requests for sick notes and medical reports are common in general practice. Dealing with these inappropriately and being judgemental in either direction may have far-reaching consequences. For example, it can result in some patients not receiving benefits to which they are entitled, or in others obtaining unfounded financial support and confirmation of their sick role. Always make sure that you know the purpose of a certificate, and try to get all the facts right. If you have to refuse a sick note, be honest with your patient and explore other ways of helping them. Offer to discuss the problem, and consider referring them for a second opinion if you are unsure whether a medical problem is genuine.

Using written messages for your patient to take home

Some patients do not like leaving without a prescription in their hands. A useful way around this is to explain your reasons for not prescribing tablets, and instead to write down a 'personal management plan'. For example, jot down general health advice for the treatment of backache or sore throats with specific advice that your patient could try first next time the problem occurs, before making an appointment. Often this does not take very long, and it sometimes appears to reduce the number of repeat consultations. Some practices also have patient information leaflets loaded on their computers so that copies can easily be printed, or you could hand out the relevant leaflets from your filing cabinet and underline the information that is relevant for that particular patient. If you feel that not prescribing anything is the most appropriate action, you may want to <u>make an effort to explain</u> to the patient that absolutely <u>no treatment is required</u> and try to lower their expectations. When explaining the effects of any intervention or treatment, the acronym 'BRAN' (what are the Benefits, Risks and any Alternatives? And what happens if you do Nothing?) can help you to remember the main points to go through.

Share your difficulties with someone else

If you are <u>really struggling</u> with a patient, <u>talk</u> to one of your <u>colleagues</u> or fellow registrars about the problem. <u>Merely sharing your thoughts can be invaluable in itself.</u> Older colleagues in particular, who may have known that patient for many years, can <u>often provide new insights and interesting details</u> about your patient's history that you may not have found in the notes. These may completely change your perspective on the matter and increase your understanding of the problem.

Keep your sense of humour

Occasionally it is easy to get frustrated with some patients, despite all your best efforts. <u>Try to remain positive and even enjoy your problem patients by regarding them as a challenge,</u> and by trying to <u>appreciate the humorous side of absurd situations.</u> If you have to see a patient whom you do not particularly like, try to find some common ground to talk about, such as sports or local issues. Although you may never become close friends, it often can improve your professional relationship dramatically. If you are lucky and discover the reason responsible for making the patient such hard work, you may even be able to <u>transform your 'heartsinks' into your 'gold star patients'</u>!

Aggressive patients

Diffusing aggressive behaviour

It seems fair to say that aggressive patients and relatives are rare, although this may vary depending on the practice area. However, intimidating or violent patients can be extremely frightening and nerve-racking. It is often difficult to maintain an objective view and not to take aggression personally, as becoming aggressive is commonly a reaction to frustration, anger or guilt. Dealing with aggressive patients or relatives is a complicated area, and much thought, experience, reflection and training will be required to become confident in dealing with it. Here are just two possible approaches that you may want to try out. When faced with unexpected aggression it may help to try to distance yourself and to attempt to put your patient at ease. Rather than playing the game and responding defensively or aggressively, see whether you can surprise your patient by being extremely polite (which admittedly is not an easy thing to do, but may sometimes be astonishingly effective!). Always think about your own and your staff's security first, and summon help quickly if a situation gets out of control.

Using role-play to prepare for difficult patients

Role-play can feel a little embarrassing if you have not done it before, but it is an extremely useful tool for anticipating and preparing for distressing consultations. For instance, you could try enacting difficult situations such as talking to an aggressive drug addict or a patient demanding a false sick certificate from you with your trainer or your colleagues (e.g. as part of a tutorial or on the day-release course). You can swap roles or experiment with your responses, and practising in a 'safe' environment and receiving feedback about your performance can be a great learning experience. It should also be far less intimidating than the real situation – unless your counterpart goes over the top, of course!

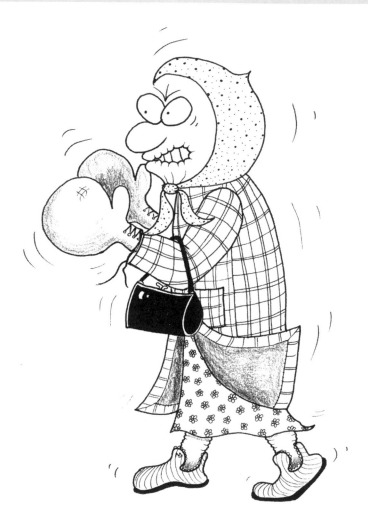

Puzzling medical problems

It is not uncommon to be confronted with symptoms or signs in your patients that either appear too mild to warrant a GP's opinion, or which do not fit any familiar picture. There are various ways to approach these 'mystery' patients that will probably be discussed as part of your training, or can be read about in more detail in books on the consultation. The following are only a couple of suggestions that can be tried initially, even with very little general practice experience.

Take trivial presentations seriously

It is very easy to become annoyed with patients who present to you with very minor symptoms. This may include parents bringing in a child who has had a mild sore throat or earache for only a few hours, at a time when you are expecting to see 'proper' emergencies. However, quite often concerns of a more serious nature may be hidden behind the façade of a minor illness, and it is worth trying to find out about any underlying concerns. For example, the mother of a child with earache may be frightened about the possibility of a diagnosis of mastoiditis from which she herself had suffered as a child. It is the parents' job to worry, but sometimes their fear may escalate out of all proportion, especially at night or if they are tired and at the end of their tether. In these cases, simple reassurance and acknowledgement of their concerns are of most help, and will be appreciated much more than a magic cure. Knowing the reasons for a patient presenting with a trivial complaint can often shed a revealing light on the issue, and being able to relieve their underlying worries can be immensely satisfying.

Approach complicated patients systematically

Patients do sometimes present with vague or difficult symptoms, and may have frequently consulted various doctors during the course of their illness. If you are unsure about what is wrong with a particular patient who is well known for consulting with non-specific complaints, it can sometimes be quite effective to start again from scratch rather than just treating individual symptoms. Reviewing the notes thoroughly, repeating a focused history, performing a comprehensive physical examination and designing a new problem list will help you to gain a new perspective, and are all particularly important if you do not know the patient very well. This is not to say that you will necessarily find out what the problem is – having to deal with uncertainty is unfortunately part of the game. However, you should be fairly reassured that you have not missed anything obvious.

Get help at a relatively early stage

When patients consult again and again with the same problem this is sometimes a sign that there is something wrong, and it should ring warning bells. The problem may be of a medical nature in that you may not have reached the full diagnosis or started appropriate treatment. Alternatively, it may have something to do with your doctor–patient relationship, and your patient may not be adequately reassured. Instead of struggling on by trying out various other treatments, try to get help whenever a patient returns more than twice with the same problem. Ask your trainer for advice and a fresh perspective, or refer your patient to another partner in the practice who may have a special interest in that particular field. However, this should be a genuine referral rather than simply dumping a problem on to someone else, so it is only polite to ask your colleague for permission first. It may be appropriate to refer your patient to a hospital specialist for a second opinion, although you should be aware of the possible effects that this may have on symptom fixation if there is no underlying physical cause. All of this should help to build a relationship of trust with your patient, and should not be seen as an admission of defeat on your part.

Children

Talk to small babies

Examining newborn babies is usually great fun. However, if they start to cry because they are unhappy for some reason, this can become rather distressing not only for them but also for the parent and yourself. Quite often babies are soothed by a gentle human voice, so talking to them softly may make examination of their heart, lungs and abdomen much easier. Moreover, accompanying individuals (usually one of the parents) will also have more confidence in you and are more likely to see you as a caring professional if you treat babies as your 'patients of honour'.

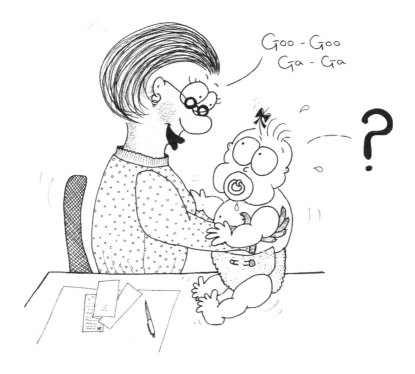

Give children time to start trusting you

Seeing children in general practice can be the highlight of your surgery – or a nightmare if they are in a bad mood. It may take a while to become confident in seeing children, and a little practice as well as patience is often required. As you only have a few minutes for each consultation, it is tempting to get down to business quickly and home in on the painful ear or throat. However, if one move is made too quickly the child can become very unco-operative, making further examination almost impossible. Children are probably more likely to trust you if their parents do so, and therefore it is usually a good idea to try to establish a rapport with the mother or father first. Talk in a calm voice and carefully establish eye contact with the child, holding back a little as soon as the child withdraws. In the case of toddlers, you might try gently touching or stroking their foot first while they are sitting on their parent's lap, which is far less threatening than immediately starting to examine them. Children in general often feel a little more at ease if you get down to their level or even below. They tend to feel vulnerable and apprehensive when lying down, and an abdomen can sometimes be felt very well with the child sitting on his or her parent's lap, or even standing in the case of older children. If a child is completely unco-operative and there is no obvious serious illness, it may be better to defer the examination and make another appointment rather than forcing the child to be examined.

Use indirect and playful language

Many children hate doing what they are told and will refuse any of your requests. However, quite often you may be able to get them interested in what you are doing. For example, if a child does not want to open his or her mouth for a throat inspection, you can ask what he or she had for breakfast. If the answer is, say, 'rice crispies', you can respond that you would like to look for some of them as proof, which may sometimes make the child open his or her mouth like a yawning lion. Looking into a teddy's or mum's ear first often helps to alleviate any fears a child may have about the auriscope. Some older children also become more co-operative if you hand over the stethoscope to them and allow them to listen to their own heart sounds.

Bring toys into the arena

It is often much easier to examine children if you can manage to distract them. Small children (and also many doctors) really enjoy playing with toys, and the more outrageous the better! You can often attract children's attention by putting some noisy wind-up toys on your desk, or attaching clip-on toys to your instruments.

For example, little monsters or 'walking dentures' are great fun for everyone involved, and can help to keep a child relaxed and attentive during your examination.

Adolescents

Be aware of potential pitfalls with adolescents

Young people who are experiencing all the ups and downs of puberty form their own group of patients that can be very rewarding but also challenging to work with. Often a fair amount of experience and training is necessary to become confident in managing all of the different problems with which adolescents present. This section can therefore only touch on this difficult area. For example, the issues of confidentiality or underage prescribing can become particularly difficult when one is dealing with adolescents requesting contraception. You will need to feel confident in this field, and should make sure that it is dealt with in sufficient detail during your training. It is relatively unusual for adolescents to present on their own in general practice, as they normally do not like going to see the doctor and are therefore usually taken there by a parent. Therefore if they come to see you alone about an apparently trivial problem, this should ring some warning bells, as there are sometimes deeper underlying reasons for making an appointment, which can be easy to miss. To mention just a few, hidden problem areas may include bullying or other problems at school, contraception or suspected pregnancy, depression, anxiety, eating problems such as anorexia nervosa and bulimia, sexual abuse and problems with parents. It is worth keeping these topics in mind and looking out for them. However, the trivial symptoms may also be completely genuine, so do not get too alarmed too soon.

Listen attentively

It is easy to regard adolescents as young adults, but in fact their position is rather unique, as they may show the conflicting attitudes and behaviour of both children and grown-ups at the same time. Try to make them feel at ease, as it may be difficult for them to talk to adults openly, and make it clear that you are listening to their point of view and are not automatically taking their parents' side. You may find that using clear and simple language mixed with humour can be a good way to avoid lecturing or sounding patronising. Often adolescents who come to see you accompanied by a parent may find it difficult to open up. Finding some excuse to send the parent out of the room for a while (e.g. asking them to check at reception when the next free appointment is available, or saying that you would like to examine their child on his or her own in your examination room) may give you an opportunity to talk to the young person alone, and may thus help him or her to be franker with you.

Record-keeping

Structure your records in the case-notes

Especially in a practice with a number of partners and non-personal lists, good communication about patients is important. As the records in general practice tend to be relatively brief, using a framework for jotting down the essential information can both help you to focus and enable others to understand your management more clearly. If your practice is fully computerised and no longer uses case-notes, find out how you can structure and highlight any of your entries. One of the most useful ways of recording is still the widely used 'SOAP' system (Subjective, i.e. complaints and symptoms; Objective, i.e. findings; Assessment and Plan). Although it is a little rigid and not necessarily appropriate for all problems encountered in general practice, it is often useful as a basic tool and starting point. In addition, it can be helpful to use problem lists liberally and to write down your views, which will make it easier for your colleagues (as well as yourself!) to follow your thoughts. It can also help to jot down what you want to do in the next consultation. This can give you a swifter start at follow-up, as it is sometimes easy to lose the plot.

Highlight important findings and test results

Time is often limited during a busy surgery, and it is difficult to review the case-notes in detail. You can make life easier for yourself and others by marking abnormal or key results with highlighted boxes, or by underlining them with a red pen. A cross-reference to any significant investigation report that has been filed elsewhere in the case-notes will also help to prevent important results being overlooked in the future.

Follow-up

Remind yourself about results that you want to look up

If you arrange investigations you may not always necessarily get to see the results yourself. This is particularly likely if you are the registrar in a practice with shared lists. One of your colleagues may look at reports while you are away, or the report may have been sent to the partner who is the registered GP for this patient. Keeping track of results is important both for your own education and also for medico-legal reasons in case you were planning to arrange follow-up. Some results may take a while to come back, and very occasionally they get lost in the post. It may therefore be useful to develop your own system of chasing up important reports that you have not seen personally.

Keep a diary for checking results

Whenever you request an important test for a patient you could write down a prospective reminder in your diary or a special calendar for follow-up. For example, if you expect a blood test report to be back in one week, make an entry in your diary for the following week stating 'Look up blood results for Mr A Nother', or something similar. When you sign reports, it is then easy to tick the entries in your diary accordingly. If a result is overdue according to your diary, at the end of the day, you could ask your receptionist to pull out the relevant case-notes for you to look at the next morning. You will then be able to check quickly whether a result has arrived and been acted upon, or whether it may need chasing up. This procedure may seem a little tedious, but in fact does not take very long at all, and will help you to keep an eye on those test results in which you are particularly interested.

Keep records of patients whom you would like to follow up

If you admit a patient as an emergency when on call, you may want to find out whether that person has recovered and whether your diagnosis was correct. Usually you will have to make a special effort, because you will not normally be informed automatically by the hospital if you work for a co-operative and see patients from other practices. One suggestion would be to keep a small notebook in your bag in which you can quickly jot down the patient's name and telephone number, your presumed diagnosis, the name of the admitting doctor and any other details. You could then write a reminder in your diary to give the hospital or family a quick ring the next day. Apart from this being very educational and full of unexpected surprises, patients and their families often really appreciate your showing an interest in what happened to them and how they are doing.

Monitor your hospital referrals

Once you have referred a patient to a specialist it may be a long time until that person is seen, and even longer until you receive a letter from the consultant. It is very easy to forget that you have referred someone after a couple of months have elapsed. In order to keep abreast with their referrals, some GPs keep a notebook on their desk in which they write down the patient's name, the date, the reason for referral and the specialist referred to as soon as they have dictated their referral. Whenever a hospital letter arrives, it is then easy to tick the relevant entry in the notebook. In this way it is possible to check at regular intervals whether a patient has been seen, and you could then try to speed things up if necessary.

Difficult home visits

Stay safe on home visits

Problems with patients or relatives on home visits are rare, but it pays to try to avoid getting into unpleasant situations, especially if you work in deprived areas. If you need to go on a potentially difficult visit, make sure that you inform your receptionists of where you are going and how long you will be away. When you are on call for a co-operative, you could ask the driver to phone you after an agreed time when seeing a problematic patient, and to call the police if you do not respond. Alternatively, you could leave the mobile phone switched on so that the driver can hear if a situation gets out of control, although this raises issues of confidentiality and may only be considered in extreme cases where your security is at great risk. Very rarely you may need to be able to leave swiftly in the event of unexpected danger to yourself, so on arrival you should consider the potential need for a quick exit. Some patients' homes may be in an appalling state, but you should try to avoid showing any signs of either disapproval or approval. Driving about in a flashy car and expensive clothes may attract unwanted attention, and swapping your doctor's bag for a rucksack may make you less obvious as a GP. Although aggression towards general practitioners is rare, assaults do occasionally occur. If you are ever attacked verbally or physically, it is absolutely essential that you talk to your trainer about it, as such an experience can be extremely disturbing and unsettling. Any form of violence towards you is completely unacceptable, and you need to get the support of your practice and colleagues. It is important that such incidents are discussed with the practice partners. If necessary, further action needs to be taken for you and your colleagues' safety, which may require involving the police.

Be very cautious in dealing with anyone under the influence of drugs or alcohol

If a patient who requests a visit sounds intoxicated on the telephone, screen the case-notes for evidence of any previous aggressive behaviour, and ask your colleagues for further details if that patient is unknown to you. Always try to obtain enough information to be sure the call is genuine and that it is safe to visit. There is often not much point in arguing with an intoxicated patient, and if a patient or relative becomes aggressive it is important to try to remain calm and not to give the impression that you are being intimidated. If the situation deteriorates further, it is often best to make your apologies, leave as soon as possible and discuss with your colleagues how to deal with and follow up this episode.

3 Talking business: communication within and outside the primary healthcare team

Using the telephone
Dictating letters
Referring to hospitals and other secondary services
Communicating with colleagues
Talking to patients' relatives
Facilitating bereavement
Handling complaints
Drug company representatives
The media
Giving evidence in court

Effective communication is one of the key skills required for working in general practice and, of course, the core element of this is your interaction with patients. However, working in primary care also entails a continuous exchange of information within the practice team and with other health professionals, and this is very important for good patient care. In addition, as a general practitioner you may have to talk to a variety of other people, such as drug company representatives or even the media. Most doctors ending their hospital training already possess all of the necessary skills required. However, it can sometimes be difficult to get your message across and to avoid loss of information when you are new to this area. To make the whole process more efficient and accurate, it may be helpful to consider adopting certain strategies that some GPs have found useful.

Using the telephone

The telephone as one of your first options

In many situations a telephone call is a much quicker and easier way of communicating than writing letters or going to see a person face to face. Whenever you are speaking to patients, relatives or hospital doctors on the phone, it is usually best to have the case-notes of the patient involved in front of you. It is only too easy to confuse patients' case histories, and by not having the necessary background information available you run the risk of getting caught out at some stage and mixing up important details, which could be a little embarrassing at the very least. Many practices are now fully computerised, and sending email messages to partners and other team members is also a very useful way of relaying certain types of message.

Prepare a structure for important telephone calls

Talking to upset relatives, an angry patient or a stressed hospital doctor can be difficult at times, and in the heat of the moment it may be easy to forget what you intended to say. Briefly running through your main arguments and jotting down the chief points you want to make before placing a call can often help you to get back on track if emotions start to run higher than expected.

Dictating letters

Learn to dictate

If you have not dictated letters before, it may take a while to get used to talking into a dictaphone, but this is certainly one of the quickest and easiest ways to produce letters. Practice is the key, and following some simple rules can greatly improve communication between you and your secretary. Most dictating machines are very similar and easy to use, but some have certain features that are worth knowing about. It is a good idea to try to scan the manual if you have a spare moment in order to find out how to make the best use of your dictaphone and obtain good recordings. By experimenting with it and listening to a sample tape on the secretary's machine you can get an idea of how your voice sounds to the typist and whether you need to adjust the volume or speed of your speech. Listening to tapes and typing letters all day can be very tedious, as many typists would readily confirm. Ask the practice secretary for some feedback on your dictation to find out whether your tapes are easy to listen to. Well-dictated tapes will help to reduce spelling mistakes and other errors, saving time and hassle for both of you. Medical secretaries often have different backgrounds and preferences, so ask them how they would like you to dictate and whether they want you to include punctuation.

Provide some basic information to brief your secretary

When starting a new tape, it is worth bearing in mind that the secretary may find it easier to identify a particular tape if you state your name and the date at the beginning. This is particularly important if you work as a locum, as she may not necessarily recognise your voice. It is also useful for the secretary to know what kind of document you are dictating (e.g. a letter, memo, certificate, etc.), as the practice may have pre-prepared templates. Special messages for your secretary are best included at the beginning of the tape. You can also attach a written note to warn of any further messages you may have added at the end that she needs to know about.

Preventing 'mix-ups' of information

When you are busy and have to dictate a number of letters, it is easy to combine the wrong case-notes with the tape accidentally (unless your practice is paperless). It is a good idea to get into the habit of stating on the tape for which patient and to whom the letter is addressed, and to attach the tape firmly to the notes by means of a strong rubber band or some similar means of preventing it from slipping off. Medical secretaries do not have a full medical training and cannot be expected to know all of the medical terms. You may spare yourself many requests for clarification if you spell difficult medical words, especially unusual drug names or those that sound similar to other words with a different meaning, and you will also reduce the number of embarrassing or sometimes even dangerous mistakes. However, it might be wise to check with the secretary first whether she minds about this, as some may be offended if you continually spell words they know. Speak slowly and clearly, and consider indicating the end of sentences by dictating 'full stop' and the end of paragraphs by stating 'new paragraph, please' to help format your letters and make them more readable, again after prior discussion.

Using standard letters

An even quicker method than dictating letters is to send out standard letters. These are often saved on the practice secretary's computer and may be useful for any type of letter that has to be written over and over again to many patients (e.g. invitations to come for review). Many practices use standard letters, and you could ask your secretary to provide you with a file of samples. You may even come up with your own idea for a standard letter, and what follows is merely a description of how it could be introduced should you get involved. You would need to agree the format and content with the other partners and consider the wording carefully. The language should be clear, factual, simple and instructive, and the letter should offer an opportunity for the addressee to respond. If you agree a code for each letter, then this and the patient's name are usually all that you need to convey to the typist so that she can print out a copy for you to sign.

Referring to hospitals and other secondary services

Provide the appropriate information

Hospital referral letters require varying amounts of detail, depending on your patient's background and the actual problem. In general, they should provide enough facts to describe the patient's condition and the context adequately. It is often easy to forget to mention even basic data when you have to dictate or write under time constraints. For this reason, having a list of paragraph titles in front of you may help you to remember all of the important topics that you might want to include in your letter. Jot down headings such as age, job, present complaint, signs, past history, drug summary, social background or investigation results, and adjust the amount of detail you provide according to the type of problem. Try also to include your line of thought, your reason for the referral and details about what you have told the patient. Clearly state (preferably as an opening gambit) what you expect from the referral (e.g. admission, advice, further investigation or taking over of management) in order to improve your chances of getting the desired result. It is usually much easier for the hospital doctor to answer a specific question than to try to guess what you are asking for. In some cases it may be more appropriate to speak directly to a consultant before you refer a patient, in order to make sure that a referral is appropriate. Many consultants will not mind talking to you on the phone, and your trainer will often be able to tell you which of the local consultants are particularly helpful.

Negotiating with hospital doctors

Occasionally you may have to haggle with an overworked hospital doctor about the need for admission of a patient, which may add to the stress that you are already experiencing while on duty. It is often difficult for junior hospital doctors to appreciate fully the difficulties that general practitioners face in the community, where it is frequently impossible to make a full diagnosis or to observe a patient as well as if they were in hospital. However, it is your responsibility to decide whether a patient needs to be admitted, and once you have made that decision you should be prepared to argue your case competently.

Anticipating questions

It will make the referral smoother and strengthen your case if you can anticipate the questions that you are likely to be asked by the hospital team and have the answers at your fingertips. For example, you should try to ensure that you have all the necessary patient details in front of you. It helps to have available the results of essential observations supporting the need for admission (e.g. all the vital signs and any positive findings). Aim to be certain in your own mind why you want that patient to be admitted, and be open about it. Even your own uncertainty or parents' anxiety or inability to cope with a sick child can be very valid reasons for seeking admission.

Stay calm and in control

Very rarely it may be necessary to argue quite strongly if your decision to admit a patient is not met with the same enthusiasm. Always be open to suggestions – after obtaining advice from the hospital team you may even agree that a patient can be safely treated or observed at home, or that they can be seen at the next appointment in the outpatient department. However, you are acting on behalf of your patient and are responsible for your actions. It is sometimes necessary to be assertive once you have made up your mind that admission is unavoidable. Refuse to be pressurised into arranging investigations that would not alter your management in an emergency, and do not be hesitant about asking to speak to a senior hospital doctor such as a registrar or consultant if you are still not getting anywhere.

Communicating with colleagues

Working in general practice once you are a little more experienced requires a great deal of independence and the ability to work on your own. It is therefore easy to feel isolated at times, especially if you are going through a slightly difficult or hectic period. The amount of contact and interaction between partners varies from one practice to another, and in addition to sharing information, meeting up with others in the practice is important for providing mutual support and understanding.

Sharing breaks with your partners

Having short breaks with your colleagues, even if only for a quick cup of coffee, can provide a good opportunity to unwind and improve the team spirit. Even if you are busy, try to make an effort to meet up with your team if you have regular, scheduled breaks. Many of the minor problems that affect the practice can often be resolved quickly and informally over a relaxed chat before they have a chance to grow and become a burden. Moreover, talking about personal matters can also make you and others more aware of any problems at home that may be causing stress at work. Knowing about any difficult periods in the personal life of a colleague may make it easier to provide support, and can ease some of the workload for the affected person at an early stage. If, due to local circumstances, you do not regularly bump into colleagues during a normal working day, why not suggest introducing informal breaks at mutually convenient times to give people a chance to meet? You should check this with your trainer first, as there may be good reasons why your colleagues decided not to meet regularly.

Asking your trainer for advice

Registrars in general practice often need to ask their trainer for a second opinion or for guidance with regard to clinical problems, especially during the first few months of training. In order to reduce waiting times to a minimum, many registrars and their trainers agree on a mutually acceptable system for contacting each other. This will very much depend on personal preference, as some trainers may like to be telephoned and interrupted during a consultation, whereas others would prefer you to wait until after they have finished seeing a patient. Try to agree on the best way to make contact. For example, you could use a coded rhythm of knocking on the door so that your trainer knows that you need advice. You can then return to your room and need not wait outside the door, as you know that your trainer will attend to your problem shortly. Allowing your surgeries to overlap with some of your trainer's administration sessions can also help to keep disruption of consultations to a minimum, as it is usually much less disruptive to interrupt paperwork.

Contacting other members of the practice team

As outlined in the first chapter, in general practice you work in a team with a wide variety of other health professionals. Find out early on how and when to contact individual team members, and try to be sensitive to their ways of working. It is useful to know the type and quantity of information that you will need to provide with your referrals, and whether there are special referral forms or communication books in the practice. A good knowledge of your colleagues' range of expertise and treatment facilities can also help to make your referrals more appropriate and sensible. If you have any special experience in certain areas (e.g. if you have worked as a paediatric registrar, have knowledge of accupuncture or speak a foreign language), do not forget to mention this, so that the team can make use of your skills as well.

Talking to patients' relatives

Identify a key person

Having to cope with a group of concerned and anxious relatives can be difficult when one of their loved family members has fallen ill. Whenever possible, ask your patients for permission regarding the passing on of any medical details to their next of kin. Always be aware of the issue of confidentiality, which may play an important role when, for example, both husband and wife are your patients or if you work in a small community where many of your patients know each other. Should you ever be in a dilemma and not know how to proceed with regard to confidentiality, try to discuss this with your trainer or other senior colleagues if you can, as in some cases breaches of confidentiality may have major implications. If you have to deal with a number of relatives, it may make communication easier if you ask the parties involved to nominate a single person through whom you will relay any important messages, otherwise it can be very easy to generate confusion among the family. Try to facilitate communication between family members, because it is important for them to be able to support each other as well.

Take relatives' requests to talk to you seriously

Whenever a relative wishes to speak to you about one of your patients, try to find some time to discuss any matters of concern. Relatives often play a central role for patients, and their worry can easily transfer on to the patient. They can be valuable informants, especially with regard to the elderly, and often provide important clues as to what is really wrong with your patient. By being available to talk to relatives of patients in nursing homes, and by being willing to discuss any of their concerns, you can also often diffuse potential grounds for complaint or suspicion. Be careful if relatives ask you not to mention to your patient that they have requested a visit. It is sometimes easy to trap yourself in a web of lies if your patient is unaware of this and you visit under false pretences. In the long term it is usually a much better idea to try to find out why a relative does not want your patient to know about their request, and not to promise anything. An air of openness and honesty is much more likely to improve the relationship with both your patient and the relative in the long term. If it is relevant and appropriate, it is good practice to record in your patient's case-notes the details of any conversations that you have had with the relatives. This will help to remind you and others at a later stage what relatives have been told, and the information may also become important for medico-legal reasons.

Bear in mind the effects of your actions on carers of the elderly or patients with physical or mental impairment

Without the help of informal carers many dependent patients would not be able to continue living in the community. Even if the care of your patient is one of your main concerns, the health of the carers is just as important, as this may directly affect your patient. Depression is very common among carers, and it can be very rewarding if on detecting signs of this you are able to take appropriate action. Financial difficulties often cause additional worries, and help with obtaining benefits that are available can significantly improve your patient's circumstances.

Facilitating bereavement

Handling a death among your patients can be quite difficult whether you are new to general practice or an experienced GP. There are many different ways of dealing with bereavement, and facing grieving patients or relatives often causes anxiety and distress in doctors as well. However, helping a family through such a difficult time can lay the foundation for an immensely improved relationship.

Acknowledge your own feelings

We all have our own personal experiences of death of relatives or friends that affect our relationship with bereaved families. The essence of general practice is to get involved with patients, and if you have looked after a terminally ill patient for a while and they have just died, this is bound to cause emotional upheaval in yourself as well as in the family. Try to acknowledge your own distress, and do not be afraid to cry with the family if your emotions suddenly take over. This is perfectly acceptable and will in no way show any weakness on your part, but merely compassion, which is often very much appreciated by the family of the patient.

Provide basic information

If you offer a list of undertakers and other practical information, as well as the addresses of bereavement counsellors in your local area, this is often welcomed by relatives. Agencies such as Age Concern, the Citizens Advice Bureau or Cruse, as well as widow and widower clubs, can often help in coping with loss, and many practices keep the leaflets and addresses of such organisations.

Explain the death certificate

Knowing the cause of death is often very important for the next of kin, and relatives often worry about a diagnosis. You can try to prevent any negative feelings in the relatives by going through the death certificate in detail. Take special care to explain the reasons for a post-mortem examination if this is or was required, as this is commonly the subject of myths and false beliefs. You can often affirm your openness by providing an opportunity for the relatives to ask questions and by leaving the envelope unsealed.

Be available to the relatives and the coroner

Many questions only arise after some time, and offering to speak to distressed relatives can alleviate a great deal of anxiety. It is equally important to agree to speak to the coroner promptly should you be contacted, in order to avoid any unnecessary delays. It is advisable to be aware of possible disputes over wills within families, and to avoid becoming involved in such arguments if possible.

Respect the family's right to privacy

There is often a very fine line between care and intrusion, and as a result it may be difficult to know how much help to offer. Most families usually appreciate a bereavement visit, but it is probably good practice to ask for permission to make such a visit beforehand. If you did not know the deceased person very well, a telephone call offering your condolences and support may be more appropriate for some families. Regardless of whether you visit or talk to the family on the phone, you may prevent problems by finding out whether a support network is available and aiming to make constructive suggestions if help is required. Even if a death was expected and the person who died was very old, it is still often a sad loss for the family. For this reason, beware of making any insensitive remarks, and try to respect the relatives' feelings.

Keep records of recent deaths

It is very important that everyone in the surgery knows of any death that has occurred in the practice area, so that all contacts with the families can be handled sensitively. Most practices put up a list or keep a book of terminally ill and recently deceased patients in an easily visible place in the main office, and it is worth looking at this every day to keep up to date. Unless this is done routinely by someone else, it is good practice to let the hospital know about a recent death, as outpatient appointments sent to a deceased person can be very upsetting for the family. Writing the cause of death according to the death certificate in the deceased patient's notes as well as in the partner's notes, together with the patient's first name, can help you to clarify any points with the partner in later consultations.

Handling complaints

Reacting to complaints

Patients tend to be more informed about medical problems these days, and may have a lower threshold for filing complaints if they consider that some aspect of their management has been unsatisfactory. This does not usually happen very often. Although sometimes a complaint may be justified, some people tend to complain more out of frustration, and it is easy to feel offended and personally attacked in such cases, which can be threatening and quite upsetting. However, complaints also provide invaluable feedback, and it is important for you to know whether patients or relatives are unhappy with any aspect of your management, for whatever reason. Most complaints are not necessarily a criticism against you personally, but rather an action arising from uncertainty, anger, worry or helplessness, so be prepared to expect complaints at any time in your professional career, even if you have not made any mistakes, and try to avoid knee-jerk reactions.

Obtaining the necessary background information

When you receive a complaint, it is sometimes best not to comment on anything before you know all the details of the case. All surgeries are obliged to have an in-house complaints procedure, and you should find out early on in your training who needs to be approached in the event of a complaint, and how the procedure works. Complaints are dealt with at various levels, and are often handled by the practice manager or a senior partner initially.

Being open and frank

We all make mistakes, and it is important to be able to admit these both to ourselves and to our patients. Many formal and informal complaints can be avoided by taking the time to find out exactly what has gone wrong. Often a simple apology or explanation early on is all that is needed and, contrary to common belief, this does not increase your risk of being sued. If you are accused of having made a mistake, it is important that you get support from others. Talking to your trainer and senior colleagues as well as to your peers about any mishaps can help you to gain an objective view and can also provide you with enormous support. If an allegation is of a more serious nature, contact your medical defence organisation early on, as they are usually more than happy to give advice over the telephone on how to deal with a particular complaint.

Drug company representatives

Making use of your time when talking to drug representatives

Undoubtedly your receptionist will regularly ask whether you could spare a few minutes to talk to a pharmaceutical company representative. Due to time constraints and fear of getting behind schedule it is often tempting to find a quick excuse and not to bother talking to them. However, talking to drug reps can be very worthwhile, but only if you are able to stay in control and know beforehand what you expect from them.

Guiding the conversation

Drug reps can provide valuable information about new drugs and developments, and are often able to produce reprints of new or landmark studies as well as educational material. Refuse politely but assertively if you do not want to hear about a drug that you already know or that is irrelevant to your practice. Trial evidence often gives you a better idea of the usefulness of a drug than glossy brochures. The drug rep should be able to quote you the three most important trials providing evidence for the efficacy of the drug. You could use the conversation as a 'critical appraisal exercise' and

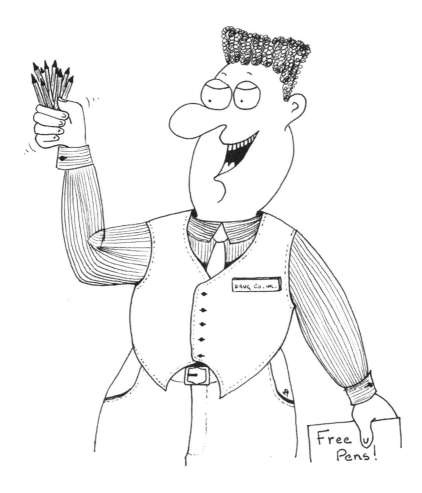

prepare yourself for asking questions on study methodology, cost-effectiveness, side effects and similar areas. Cultivating critical awareness will help you to find out how much and what kind of evidence is backing the promoted drug, and in addition it is good preparation for the MRCGP examination. It is often best not to say that you prescribe a drug when you do not, as you can easily be found out via the pharmacy. You may also want to consider some guidelines for yourself with regard to accepting any gifts, and err on the side of caution if anything seems 'over the top'.

The media

Expecting requests for information from the media

Today's media are on the whole very interested in health topics, and new medical developments and local or national medical disasters quickly make the headlines of newspapers and television programmes. Although it is unlikely that a journalist will ever select you for an interview, it may not be such a remote possibility in the case of a local event involving your practice or one of your patients. As you are likely to be inexperienced in talking to journalists, this can be potentially very embarrassing and may cause you sleepless nights. There may also be a small risk that you accidentally provide information that you should have handled more sensitively.

Responding to journalists

Do not ignore enquiries from reporters, as they are likely to report the story anyway, with or without your help. It is very easy for them to assume that you have something to hide if you are consistently unavailable. It is usually a good starting point to find out to whom you are talking and whether that person is a specialist medical reporter or a general journalist. Try to find out what their questions are and the name of their employer or agent. You could then offer to ring them back after having consulted your colleagues, so that you can make some preparatory notes about what you wish to say.

Following simple rules of journalism

It is generally wise to be cautious about what you say to reporters, as everything will be on the record unless you agree otherwise. Any journalist is free to quote everything you say and to mention your name. It is therefore a good idea to get any replies right first time and not to comment on any issues or publications that you do not know much about or have not seen. Try to respect exclusive stories

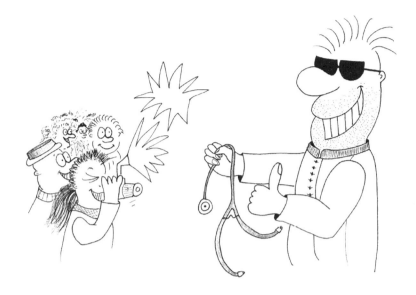

and aim to answer questions concisely. Sometimes there may be a significant difference of opinion between journalists and doctors about what is newsworthy, which can be very difficult to accept if it arises unexpectedly. If you have realistic expectations then you may avoid being disappointed, as it is very unlikely that you will be able to see the story before it appears in print.

Making your own news

Establishing contact and rapport with your local newspaper or radio and television station can raise your practice profile. It can also help to publicise new campaigns in your practice area, or new referral schemes, and can generally raise awareness of practice issues in the community. However, as these are areas that concern the whole practice, it is best to discuss any contact with the local media with your trainer and the other partners beforehand.

Giving evidence in court

Fortunately the need to appear in court or at an inquest does not often occur, and most GPs never have to answer questions before a judge or coroner during their professional life. However, inquests into deaths do occur regularly and may involve one of your patients. Even if you were not directly involved or to blame for anything, you may still be required to give evidence. Patients are now more likely to sue, and being grilled by a barrister can be both nerve-racking and unsettling. However, appearing in court can also be an interesting and informative experience so long as you follow a few simple rules.

Prepare yourself emotionally

Being questioned by a judge or lawyer can feel very threatening. Most doctors who are put on the spot feel rather anxious, and it helps to prepare thoroughly before appearing in court. Contact your medical defence organisation early on, as they can often provide useful advice and helpful printed information.

Anticipate questions about your management

Inquests into deaths are reasonably common, and may occur many years after an incident. As it is impossible to remember all your patient contacts, it can probably not be overemphasised how important it is to try to keep clear, accurate and legible notes, and also to time and date every entry. To some this may sound a little obsessive, but it may prove crucial, especially when treating acute medical conditions, when thorough documentation of the exact timing of events can be greatly in your favour. Whenever you write anything in your patient's notes, it may help to bear in mind that at some stage your lines may be read out in court, which could be rather embarrassing if you have made any flippant or inappropriate remarks.

State your evidence clearly

Your primary role in an inquest is to describe your findings and management in plain English to non-specialists, and to help them to reach a conclusion. It is best to try not to mix facts and opinion, and also expect to have to justify what you have done. Critical questioning by the lawyers is part of the process of testing evidence, and by reading your statement carefully you can often anticipate likely questions and work out how you would answer them in advance.

Answer questions appropriately

In the heat of the moment it may be very easy to get sidetracked in your explanations. Listening to questions carefully and confining your answers to precisely what was asked can be more difficult than expected when you are being put on the spot. It usually helps all non-medically qualified individuals present if you do not use technical terms without explaining them. Aim to speak slowly and clearly, and address the judge – not the defence lawyer who asked the questions. Although you may be asked provocative questions, try not to argue with the barrister or lose your temper, and try to avoid offering your opinion unless you are asked for it. Remember that in most cases you are neither being blamed nor considered an expert in all fields, so there is no harm in stating that you do not feel competent enough to answer a particular question that falls outside your area of expertise. Being straightforward and truthful but not vague about anything generally tends to be the safest option.

4 Rushing about: time management in general practice

Starting your day

Saving time during surgery sessions

Dealing with paperwork

Meetings

Home visits

The pace of a normal working day in general practice can resemble anything from a gentle stroll to a roller-coaster ride – depending on circumstances such as time of year, practice area and absent partners. Most of us learn to cope with these sudden changes in work intensity during our hospital training. However, general practice presents an additional challenge, as a larger number of decisions – whether trivial or life-saving – occasionally have to be made quickly and often under time pressure. Sometimes a certain amount of skill is required to deal with these demands and interruptions effectively. Telephone calls, requests from the receptionist, busy surgeries and administrative paperwork all force you to manage your time in the best possible way. Some very basic time-saving techniques can be invaluable, and will reduce the likelihood that you will miss your lunch break or an engagement in the evening, but probably the greatest benefit of good time management is to have more quality time both with your patient and for yourself.

Starting your day

Set priorities for your activities

Working in general practice may require you to be able to deal with a number of different requests and demands at the same time. While seeing patients during a busy surgery, you may be asked to go on an urgent visit, speak to a drug representative, sign urgent prescriptions or talk to an angry relative on the telephone. This may sometimes be rather overwhelming, as all these requests may seem equally pressing. Whenever this situation occurs, try to sit down for a minute and quickly write down all of the jobs you have to do. Although this may seem obvious, writing down your tasks really does help you to focus better. Then decide on the urgency and importance of each job and number them all in the order in which you want to tackle them – one job at a time. It is important to be flexible about this. If a job is not particularly urgent or important, you may still want to do it before the others if there is a clear advantage to doing so. For example, signing a prescription for someone who is waiting at the reception desk or looking at a wound before the treatment-room nurse puts on a new dressing can both be done very quickly. Responding to such tasks promptly will clear your mind and enable you to concentrate on the next job. It also helps others to work effectively, as their time is valuable, too.

Deal with unpleasant tasks first

Certain tasks – such as making an overdue apology or telephoning an angry patient – can tend to fall to the bottom of the list and be put off repeatedly. Why not make it a habit to tackle the most disagreeable job first? This will give you a feeling of relief and achievement, and it may give a positive feel to the whole day, as you will already have dealt with the most difficult piece of work. Many larger jobs become much easier if they are broken down into smaller, more manageable chunks, and this is best done in writing, by jotting down each step. Even a telephone call can be approached in this manner: first look up the number and write it down, then decide on a time to make the call, review the case-notes, and plan and note down what you want to say. When you finally make the call, you will find the whole task much less of a chore.

Avoid perfectionism

High expectations and the desire to do everything perfectly are relatively common among doctors. Striving for excellence is of course desirable, but wanting to be perfect all of the time may lead to considerable time-wasting. For instance, is it really necessary to explore every minor detail in a patient's history for the sake of completeness? Does your chiropody referral actually require a lengthy and elaborate social history, which may take you half an hour to research and write down? A brief and succinct case history is often much more appropriate than an intricate account of every last detail. Compact and well-structured referral letters that contain only the relevant information can also help you to focus on the problem, and are usually much easier for the recipient to read. For most jobs it is often best to try to be concise and to the point. Generally speaking, as soon as you feel you have done a job well enough, it is time to move on to something else.

Saving time during surgery sessions

Prepare your surgery and anticipate problems

Time can become very precious once you have started a busy surgery. Most appointments are only a few minutes long, and it can be easy to fall behind schedule due to unexpected circumstances. However, many of the problems that may slow you down during a session can be anticipated. It often pays to spend 10 or 15 minutes before you start your surgery scanning quickly through your patients' case-notes. Looking at the problems discussed at the last consultation and frequently being able to guess the reason for the patient's attendance can be invaluable. For example, if a patient comes to see you after an outpatient appointment, you can make sure that you have read the consultant's letter or the test report beforehand – or get your secretary to chase them up if they are not in the notes. Thus you will be informed and can discuss the issue with your patient without having to chase around and waste valuable minutes, which will give you more quality time with your patient. The hospital consultant may have recommended starting new drugs, so you can check in advance that there are no contraindications from the patient's previous history and that there is no interaction with any pre-existing medication. Enter the new drug on the computer record, print out the prescription and sign it so that the consultation can be devoted to discussion with the patient, rather than looking up and checking the new drug for its suitability.

If it is evident from the case-notes that a patient will require an investigation, then the relevant X-ray or blood request forms can often be filled out in advance. If you were planning an invasive procedure, collect and arrange the necessary equipment beforehand so that you have enough time for a thorough explanation of what you are going to do. You can then immediately get down to business without having to look for specimen pots or the correct instruments before you start. There are often other similar pointers in the case-notes that may prompt you to sort things out in advance, and by anticipating problems and acting accordingly your surgeries will run much more smoothly.

Use your examination room

Many surgeries have separate examination rooms attached to the main consulting room. These tend to be underused, as it is often felt that moving patients in and out of the consulting room is tedious and tiresome. However, it can prove highly practicable when you are dealing with small children, frail elderly patients or other patients who need time to get dressed. Inviting them into the adjacent examination room means that they can get undressed at their own pace. You can then use this time quietly in your consulting room to do other things (e.g. print prescriptions, look up references, think about your management plan, see the next patient) or just relax, go to the toilet or make yourself a cup of tea. However, you will always have the option of staying in the examination room (e.g. to watch a mother undress her baby or to assess the mobility of an elderly patient) for as long as is necessary before going back into your consulting room once you have obtained enough information.

Agree a code with the receptionist

Sometimes telephone calls can be very disruptive (e.g. when you are performing an intimate examination, or in the middle of a difficult consultation). Most practices have a policy with regard to interruptions, and it is worth finding out about this. However, if there appears to be a problem, it might be an idea to raise the issue in one of the practice meetings in order to decide whether some rules need to be agreed with the receptionists and other staff. One possibility would be to ask the receptionist not to disturb any of the partners, and to leave a message in the in-tray if the doctor's phone is not being answered after four or five rings. This way the receptionist will know that you are busy but will attend to the problem swiftly as soon as you have a spare moment. You will also know that the phone will stop after one or two rings (and you can turn the volume down if necessary), so you can get on with what you are doing. Alternatively, a special 'phone time' can be agreed after morning surgery. To prevent confusion, it is often best for individual doctors not to have separate arrangements with the receptionist, but to agree a common policy.

Dealing with other interruptions

Various requests from patients and practice staff may result in interruption of surgeries, and these can be annoying and irritating if they appear to disturb the flow of the consultation or cause delay. However, interruptions need not always be inconvenient, as they may enable you to deal very quickly with certain matters that would take up much more of your time if they were left until later. For example, answering a telephone call from a patient seeking advice between consultations may prevent problems and could save you a home visit later. Or if the treatment-room nurse asks you to take a blood specimen from a patient with 'difficult' veins, she may be very happy to get everything ready and even offer to clear away the equipment afterwards if you are accommodating and willing to interrupt a busy surgery. In this way you will save time for everyone involved and will not have to deal with an extra appointment at the end of the session. If your secretary asks you to send some urgent information about a patient to the hospital, she may be prepared to do some of the necessary research and photocopying for you or to make further phone calls if necessary. Similarly, other minor jobs can often be delegated immediately to the interrupting person and thus save you time.

Dictate letters during consultations

Dictating a pile of letters after surgery can be tiresome, as you may already have forgotten some details of the consultations and have to refresh your memory by going through the case-notes again. Longer and more complicated letters need to be left until you have finished your session, but some of the shorter ones can often be dictated in front of the patient during the consultation. This may have the advantage that facts regarding the patient's past history, current circumstances and symptoms can be clarified immediately. You can also gently reinforce certain health messages (dictating, for example, 'I have advised him/her to stop smoking in the meantime . . .' while glancing at the patient) and appear efficient by dealing with the referral promptly. You will also build up the patient's trust, and if the referral takes a while to process, at least both of you will know that you have done your part. Letters will automatically be more concise and to the point, as time is limited during the consultation and other patients will be waiting.

Save time between consultations

Many consulting rooms are situated at the end of a long corridor. If you have to call in patients personally, this can take up valuable minutes which add up substantially over the months. It might therefore be useful to suggest at one of the practice meetings the possibility of installing an electronic calling system. Many GPs like to call in their patients personally, but if the distance between waiting area and consulting room is considerable, using a calling system may be the best option. You may not want to use it all the time if you prefer the exercise, and getting out of your room after a consultation can help to clear your mind, but it will be very useful if you are busy and have trouble keeping up with your workload. Another option is to provide a second waiting area outside your consulting room with only a couple of chairs. Your next patient can be sent by the receptionist to wait outside your consulting room while your current patient is already with you, although a completely soundproof consulting room is essential in this case to maintain patient confidentiality.

Improve the techniques you use to end a consultation

If you are running late and have to deal with a particularly chatty patient, you sometimes need to be able to end a consultation swiftly without appearing to be rude. The following are only a few of the various options available that could be chosen and about which you will learn more on the day-release course when talking about consultation technique. Often an honest comment such as 'I am sorry, but I really must get on now' is all that is required. You can also try to summarise the consultation and clarify the situation by saying 'I think that's about as far as we can get today. Why don't we continue at your next appointment?'. Non-verbal communication may also help you to convey the message that the consultation is about to finish, for instance by starting to sign the case-notes and putting them back into the folder. If this does not have the desired effect, slowly get up from your chair and continue the discussion while standing. You could then help your patient into their coat and slowly open the door. By this stage most people will have realised that the end of the consultation is imminent, and you will then be able to see your next patient. Only very rarely would this be perceived as impolite behaviour.

Delegate tasks

The roles of general practitioners are expanding, and the ability to delegate has become increasingly important for freeing up time needed for tasks that only you can do. A first step is to consider whether there are parts of your work that could be done more effectively by someone else. Again, it is important to find out about the practice culture in this respect. As a registrar you should probably talk to your trainer or another partner first if you want to delegate work to someone else. If you do most of your photocopying yourself, find out whether this is something that the secretaries or receptionists in your practice would normally do. Also check out the procedures in which the practice nurse has been trained (e.g. ear-syringing or taking cervical smears). However, before you start to delegate any of the clinical procedures, make sure that you learn how to do them properly yourself and keep up your skills, as you will need them when you are on your own or if you later work in other practices with different policies. Delegation does not mean dumping work on others, but rather making the best use of everyone involved and enhancing others' jobs. There-fore, if you are ever asked to help in organising delegation in your practice, try to make the whole process of delegation as smooth as possible by following a set routine. First, decide which tasks to delegate and discuss this with the other partners and staff involved. If a suitable person is available, find out whether he or she is prepared to take on the work. Then write a simple protocol and train the member of staff. This only takes a few moments for a simple job, but may involve detailed instructions and training with supervision for more complex tasks such as clinical procedures. Finally, check how everyone involved is coping with the arrangement, and reward the extra effort. Be supportive to those to whom you delegate, and explain how you are trying to make full use of everyone's skills. Often people will be much more inclined to help if you can get them interested and involved in the change that you are proposing.

Try to keep non-attenders to a minimum

Many practices experience difficulty in providing enough appointments, which can be partly due to patients who fail to turn up. This is both a waste of resources and can make your surgeries run longer. Minor degrees of non-attendance are probably unavoidable, but if the practice is pressed for appointment times and patients regularly fail to turn up, you may want to try to tackle the problem. If someone in your surgery keeps an eye on the numbers of non-attenders, assist with the monitoring by reporting patients who fail to attend, and make a record of this in the case-notes. At the next appointment you can then remind them to cancel their appointment at short notice rather than just not turning up, as their slot can almost always be given to someone else instead. However, once a patient has failed to turn up, there is not much you can do at this stage apart from seizing a good opportunity for a quick cup of tea or a little relaxation.

Dealing with paperwork

Develop a system of filtering and organising your mail

Most general practitioners receive a substantial number of letters and publications through the post every day, and unless dealt with promptly these may easily accumulate and mount up to form an unmanageable heap of paper. Many practices arrange for either the secretary or the receptionist to screen the incoming mail for general information and advertisements that can be filed and then made available to all doctors in a float file. Unless you clear your tray very often, you could ask them to mark letters that require urgent attention or to put them into a separate tray. You could also suggest having the mail processed as much as possible. For example, certain forms can be at least partly filled in before they reach you, automatically accompanied by the relevant case-notes where necessary.

Process your mail quickly

Many GPs aim to clear their in-tray every day, as it is usually much easier to keep on top of it rather than to have to catch up all the time. If you regularly accumulate a large paper mountain it may be an idea to include a special 'clearing session' in your timetable every week in order to get rid of it as quickly as possible. You may also save some time by throwing anything of little relevance straight into the wastepaper basket, and developing a filing system that makes sorting and retrieval of written information easy. In general, try to deal with 90% of your paperwork at first pass. If you want to, you can check how well you are doing by applying the 'red-dot technique', which involves marking each piece of paper with a red dot every time you handle it in order to see how many documents accumulate more than the desired single red point.

Arrange for your mail to be processed while you are on holiday

Many practices have an agreed way of dealing with each other's mail while colleagues are away, and the receptionist or your trainer will be able to tell you how the system works. For example, you could pair up with another partner and cover each other while one of you is away, or distribute the mail of the absent person among everyone else. This avoids important matters being delayed,

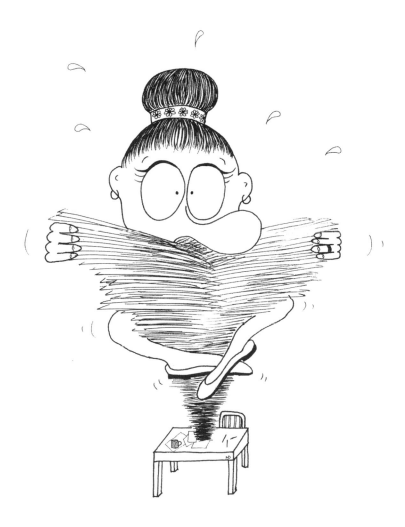

maintains the smooth running of the practice and, of course, you will not have to face the prospect of an overflowing and depressing in-tray on your return to work. However, sometimes it can be a disadvantage not to have seen the mail. For this reason, ask your partners to arrange for copies to be made of important letters or results addressed to you before they get filed away, and to put them in your mailbox. Set aside one or two hours for reading these on the morning of your return, and you will be able to catch up on what has happened during your absence.

Sign prescriptions efficiently

Signing prescriptions can form a substantial part of the daily paperwork. Even if a prescription has been generated on the computer, always check the details yourself before you sign, as you may be held responsible for any mistakes. Try to find out what rules your practice has established with regard to repeat prescriptions. Unless an established system is already in place in your practice, check regularly how many repeat prescriptions have been issued without review, and invite the patient to make an appointment if you are unsure whether a particular drug is still required. If a patient's various tablets always run out at different times, ask him or her to bring in all medication at the next appointment. You can then try to synchronise these (e.g. by making use of the 'Number of days' slot on the prescription form). By amending the quantity to be supplied, the total number of prescriptions that have to be issued can often be reduced. The time needed to change medications to repeats on the computer is usually time well spent.

Drug monitoring

Some drugs require regular review and monitoring. Many practices therefore only supply medication for a maximum of four to eight weeks. The office staff are often asked to highlight every repeat prescription for reauthorisation after a certain period (e.g. every tenth repeat or so – this is sometimes already done automatically by the practice computer) and to add the case-notes to the prescription on these occasions. In this way it will be easy to check on the last consultation and the need for continued treatment. Try to use this opportunity to screen the latest laboratory reports and arrange a blood test if necessary. Writing a quick letter or making a phone call asking patients to attend for review of their medication and symptoms if they have not been seen recently also does not take long. It helps to avoid medication errors and also reduces the number of unnecessary prescriptions.

Make the best use of your spare time

Quite often gaps will appear during your working day, which can become quite irritating if you start to wait around impatiently. It is helpful to have pending paperwork available for these unexpected waiting periods. For example, you could sign a few prescriptions or letters while waiting for a patient to arrive, or you could take your unread mail or a medical insurance report that needs to be filled in along to practice meetings if these do not start on time for any reason, thereby transforming potentially annoying waiting periods into welcome opportunities. A wonderful alternative is simply to relax and have a cup of tea.

Meetings

Make the most of meetings

Getting together can be useful for exchanging information, mutual education, reaching agreements and keeping in touch socially. However, meetings can also be time-consuming and may not always be the best way of exchanging thoughts. After a few weeks you will probably have a fairly good idea of how your practice works. Many practices review their working patterns on a regular basis and encourage registrars to make constructive comments. If you feel that there are certain aspects which could be improved in your practice, your partners may be very open to reasonable suggestions, and you should not feel shy about mentioning these. Reviewing how you work and communicate is an important aspect of being a GP, so there is no reason why you should not start to become involved in this early on as a registrar.

Stay in control

To prevent meetings from going on for ever, you may suggest agreeing fixed starting and finishing times with everyone and making an effort to adhere to them. Moving the weekly practice meetings from a mid-week lunchtime slot to Monday morning can also make them more productive, as everyone's mind should be relatively clear after the weekend, so they may be better able to concentrate on the issues being discussed. It will also be in everyone's interest to finish on time before the first patients arrive. Many of the topics discussed can then be dealt with during the week, and the main meeting will be out of the way. It often helps to have a leader (usually the practice manager) and an agreed agenda. To keep track of plans and decisions, it can be useful to document the main results by routinely asking someone to write down the minutes and keeping them in a file for future reference.

Home visits

As a registrar you will learn a lot about your patients and their social environment when you visit them at home, and this is a wonderful opportunity to get an impression of how the local practice community lives. Home visits can be full of surprises, giving unexpected insights into your patients' lives, and may be very enjoyable. However, on very hectic days they may take up a lot of time that you would sometimes rather spend at the surgery.

Routine visits

When looking objectively at home visits, it is sometimes clear that many of these visits are not essential at all, and that the interval between the visits could be safely increased. Many patients on the list for regular review improve during the course of their illness and could come up to the surgery once they have regained their mobility or are able to drive again. Many visits do not necessarily need a doctor for review. Another member of the practice team (e.g. the community nurse or health visitor) can in selected cases perform an assessment much more appropriately, provided that you agree to visit immediately yourself should there be any unforeseen problems. Some practices have drawn up guidelines on how to deal with hospital discharges and chronic or terminal illnesses in order to make visiting within the practice more consistent. However, opinions with regard to home visits vary, and it should be up to individual doctors to visit more frequently if they feel that this is necessary. A good way to prevent wasted journeys is to phone the patient before you leave to check that they are at home, especially if they live far away.

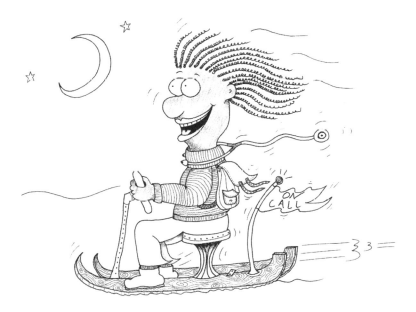

Urgent visit requests

Try to encourage patients to come and see you at the surgery, unless you feel for any reason that you would rather see someone at home. Spending some time asking detailed questions about the symptoms and development of the condition over the phone will often give you a fairly accurate idea of the relative urgency of the call. Many urgent cases do not necessarily require a visit, and diagnostic and therapeutic equipment is often more readily available at the surgery. However, in order to persuade patients to come to the surgery, you need to provide quick access as well as thorough and adequate explanation on the telephone. Agreeing to see patients immediately for an urgent problem usually takes far less time than a home visit and is less disruptive. Many parents can be reassured that there are only a few occasions when it is unsafe to bring a child to the surgery. Some out-of-hours visit requests, especially over a weekend, can often be anticipated and pre-empted by a little forward planning. Whenever possible, try to reassure your patient or their relatives by explaining the likely course of an illness, and by giving advice on how to deal with complications. It is also important for them to know exactly what constitutes a real emergency, and when to call for medical advice or an ambulance immediately. In areas of low car ownership, encourage your patients to plan in advance how they could get to the surgery, if necessary by involving their neighbours, friends or relatives. In addition, prescribing enough medication to last over a weekend or bank holiday can help to reduce the number of additional visit requests and extra work considerably.

Helping each other

When you are on daytime emergency duty, you will regularly be called out to make an urgent visit, and it may be some time before you are able to come back and continue your surgery. If you were scheduled to have any booked appointments during that period, many practices have developed strategies for dealing with waiting patients in the mean time, to avoid developing a backlog. For example, patients can be told that you are going to be delayed and could be offered the option of either waiting for you or having another appointment later that day or in the near future, whichever they prefer. An alternative is for the receptionist to distribute some of the scheduled patients equally among the other partners until you are back, or to reduce the number of extra patients for you at the end of surgery. It is good practice always to let your receptionist know where you are going and how long you expect to be out of the surgery, so that they can plan accordingly.

5 Staying calm: how to cope with stress in surgery

Techniques for reducing stress

Stress during surgeries

Implementing change

Most training practices provide a gentle introduction for new registrars with longer appointments and shorter surgeries. The amount of paperwork, emergency duties, home visits and interruptions will initially be very small compared to the workload of established partners, so the first few weeks in general practice will usually be fairly peaceful. However, this situation tends to change once your clinical responsibility has started to increase. Despite supervision and back-up from your trainer and the other partners, as time goes by you will have to make more and more important decisions on your own, and as your surgeries get busier, it may sometimes be difficult to make confident and quick decisions under pressure.

Stress levels can be high merely due to the fact that we perceive what we do as stressful. On some days even moderate workloads may bother us, while on others every minor disruption seems annoying. A certain amount of stress is probably both important and necessary to keep us going. It is well known that the popularity of adventure holidays and many extreme sports is at least partly due to the 'kick' they provide by putting people under some kind of stress. In a similar way, a busy and 'buzzing' day in general practice can be very invigorating and produce an exciting sense of alertness. However, the balance can easily tip, with too much stress causing distress and leading to a feeling of loss of control. Work then becomes a struggle, and you may find that you suddenly become less productive than you would like to be.

Techniques for reducing stress

Face conflict

Most practices are pleasant to work in, and registrars are usually made to feel very welcome. However, you may find that you do not get on with one or more members of the practice team. This could be a receptionist, the nurse, the practice manager or even your trainer. If you feel that this is the case, it may be an idea to talk to that person early on to try to identify the problem. However, this is often easier said than done, and talking to your friends or colleagues may help you to shed new light on the situation, or may even suggest a solution. Very rarely, personality clashes may be of a more serious nature and, particularly if this involves your trainer, you probably ought to discuss the situation with your course organiser or regional adviser in confidence. Changing your training practice could be one option if all else fails.

Get to know your personal reactions to stress

When you are looking after patients and dealing with extensive and complicated medical or social problems, it is very easy to become so completely absorbed in your work that you neglect your own health. It is important to recognise symptoms of too much stress in yourself, and becoming unusually irritated with patients, feeling depressed, starting to drink more alcohol or dreading going to work could be warning signs that your batteries are starting to run low. If this happens, it may help to be self-aware and analyse yourself in the same way that you would diagnose a patient. Consider what you would advise if you found these symptoms in someone else, and if this does not improve matters consider talking to your trainer, other colleagues, friends or your own GP.

Reflect on your attitudes to work

When starting in general practice, most doctors have high expectations of themselves and try to work to high standards. This is very commendable, but it can lead to an increase in stress and anxiety if you cannot achieve the goals that you have set yourself. Set aside some time, alone or with your trainer, and consider what you would like to achieve in the short, medium and long term (*see also* Chapter 1 on starting as a registrar in general practice). Rather than listing general aims such as 'become a good GP', be specific and define aims such as 'learn guidelines for emergency contraception' or 'talk to practice nurse about how the treatment room works', but make sure that you write them down. Always try to be realistic and break down your short-term goals into bite-size chunks. If you review regularly what you have written down (perhaps with someone else, such as your trainer or a colleague), it will be fairly easy to keep track of your achievements.

Develop skills to deal with failure

Although most of us try to keep mistakes to a minimum, minor and sometimes even major mistakes do unfortunately occur from time to time and can never be completely avoided. Developing your own system of arranging follow-up can help you to deal with medical problems that you are uncertain about, and will reduce the likelihood of any major disasters (*see* Chapter 2 on effective consultations). Try talking to your trainer and other colleagues openly about mistakes that you have made (or think you have made!). It can be a tremendous relief to have someone else help to put a situation in perspective, possibly making you realise that you may not have acted wrongly in the first place. Try to learn from any mistakes you make, so that there will always be a positive side to any blunder, as no one is perfect!

Take part in significant event audit

Events such as unexpected deaths due to misdiagnosis or emergency situations in the practice that have not been dealt with appropriately can put an enormous strain on the whole practice, and may lead to feelings of inadequacy and failure among members of the practice team. All of the parties involved need support, and it is important to find out what went wrong in order to learn from any mistakes that may have been made. Significant event audit is very important for dealing with these stressful events together rather than in isolation, and you should try to encourage this in your practice if your colleagues find it difficult to address these issues.

Maintain a balance between your private and working life

Getting involved in your patients' problems can make switching off after work very difficult. If you are to enjoy your work and stay interested in your patients, regular recharging of your batteries is essential. Keeping up with your hobbies or developing new ones can help to restore the balance between your personal and working life. Spend time with and enjoy your family and friends, and do not let your working life take over completely.

Value your contacts in the practice team

Other members of the practice team can be a very useful source of support. Having a cup of coffee with one of the partners, the receptionists or the cleaners after a busy day can be very relaxing. This gives everyone the opportunity to offload, unwind and chat about issues that might otherwise be on their minds all evening. Similarly, just sitting back and spending a few minutes chatting with a friendly patient during a hectic surgery or while doing home visits can be very refreshing, and often gives you surprising insights into the patient's life.

Try not to do everything yourself

Sitting alone with patients in your consulting room can give rise to the desire to tackle every problem on your own. Do not be afraid to ask for help when a situation seems to get out of control. Members of the practice team rely on each other, and many colleagues will be very willing to help you if you become completely bogged down with work. Consider delegating jobs that could be done equally well (or better!) by someone else, and try to foster an atmosphere of mutual support in the practice, playing your part as well and offering help when your colleagues are busy.

Remember appreciative patients

Some doctors file any 'thank you' letters that they receive from grateful patients in a special folder. Far from being a form of self-congratulation, this can often be a valuable personal resource for those depressing moments when you feel that everything you do seems to go wrong. Just sitting back on your own, having a cup of tea and reflecting while reading a couple of appreciative letters in privacy can put you back on track and provide a little comfort when your spirits are low.

Have a tick-list for annoying moments

We all have our own personal 'sensitive spots' and tend to get irritated, for instance, by patients arriving late or by having to deal with more extra patients than usual. You could try keeping a tick-list in your desk to help you to cope with all those irritating occasions that you cannot do much about. Mark a tick each time something very annoying happens, and treat yourself after 10 or 20 ticks to something a little luxurious, such as a new CD or a ticket for a concert. This is sometimes very effective in limiting your anger by associating a positive outlook with your small treat. But no cheating, please!

Try to become more assertive at work

Being assertive does not mean acting aggressively or becoming pushy. On the contrary, it is a way of putting forward your own ideas, feelings and needs, and equally respecting the right of others to do the same. It also means being able to stand your ground in a non-threatening manner, which can help you to take more initiative and handle difficult situations more effectively. In addition, assertive behaviour involves learning to say 'no'. Time is often at a premium in general practice, and not being able to work at a comfortable pace can make your work very stressful. Decline invitations to lectures and meetings of doubtful benefit, where your presence is not really required, and try to avoid getting overloaded with other commitments. If you find this difficult, look out for local or national courses on how to become more assertive (seminars and workshops are sometimes organised by the BMA or the Royal College of General Practitioners and are advertised in the GP press or on their web sites). You could also browse through the business and GP section of your local bookshop, where you may find helpful ideas on assertiveness, stress at work and time management in a variety of books.

Use music to relax

It can be incredibly refreshing to lie down on your examination couch for a couple of minutes after a hectic morning surgery and listen to some of your favourite music. Perhaps you have a spare tape recorder at home that you could use for this purpose, or you could buy a relatively inexpensive new one. A little relaxation of this kind may improve your concentration noticeably for the next few hours, but everything in moderation – unless you don't mind waking up in the middle of the afternoon with a long queue of patients waiting for you! Some of the more boring paperwork can also become much more tolerable with your preferred music playing in the background.

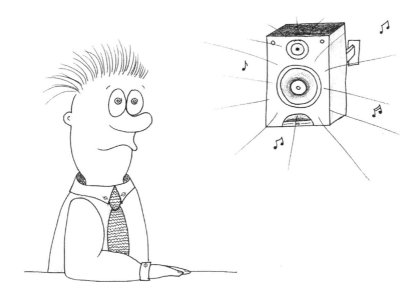

Be objective when comparing your workload with that of others

Sometimes frustration and negative feelings arise from thinking that your colleagues are dumping work on you. This may be the case, but you should be very careful about making any assumptions. Try to gather some kind of objective evidence (e.g. number of home visits or emergency appointments) before mentioning your concern to anyone. More often than not you will find that you are wrong. As a rule, if you are feeling hard done by you are probably only working just as hard as your colleagues! Moreover, any offers you may make to help a colleague on a frantic day while you are having a quiet spell will usually be very warmly received, and may be returned in the future.

Appreciate the stresses at different stages during your general practice career

It is easy to fall into a state of self-pity, but knowledge and understanding of the various pressures on yourself and your

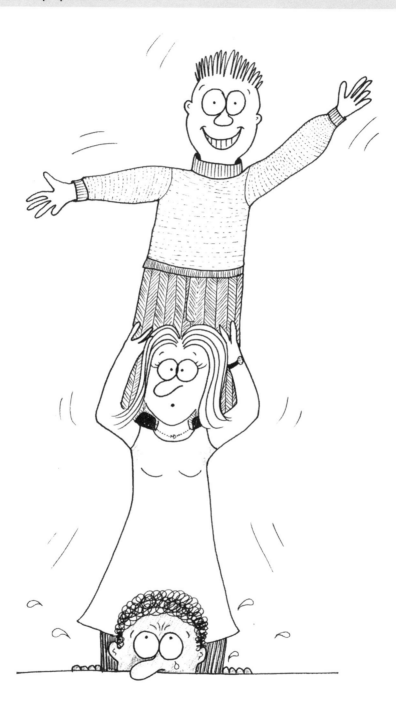

colleagues will often help to increase empathy in both directions. It is important for registrars to realise that established partners have to deal with far more paperwork and other commitments than they do. On the other hand, principals need to recognise the stresses on registrars that result from undergoing summative assessment and preparing for the MRCGP examination in addition to their clinical commitments.

Stress during surgeries

Learn to cope with delays

The time that is required for each consultation depends on various factors, including your personality and the individual problems with which patients present. For example, some doctors attract more patients with psychiatric problems, which invariably take longer to sort out than a quick succession of sore throats. Whenever you get delayed, try not to panic – even the best doctors overrun! It is far more important to provide good care for your patients than to be obsessed by keeping to time schedules. Try not to rush too much, as this will make you feel even more stressed and also more likely to make mistakes or forget things.

Identify your personally required appointment length

If you have gained a reasonable amount of experience and still find keeping to time during surgeries very difficult, you may want to explore other options if regularly running late is stressful for you. For example, you could discuss with your trainer (or, once you have qualified as a GP, the other partners in your practice) whether it would be possible to increase the length of your appointments. If you come to work early every morning in any case to avoid the rush-hour traffic, starting half an hour earlier and seeing a couple of patients in that time could prevent tension from rising during the following hours. Some patients might even prefer to see you early in the day before they have to go to work. Alternatively, you may be happy to lose half an hour of your lunch break and finish later while keeping the same number of appointments, only slightly more widely spaced. Another way of reducing pressure is to introduce 'comfort breaks' in the middle of a very long surgery in which to catch up.

Tell your patients on arrival how far behind you are

Most patients will accept the need to wait for a while if you deal with their problems adequately during the consultation. However, as with waiting for a delayed train, people usually prefer to know for how long they have to wait. If they know that you are at least half an hour behind, they may decide to go out for a stroll or make a telephone call in the mean time. If you make an announcement yourself in the waiting-room, or ask your receptionist to do this for you, your patients will usually be much less inclined to be angry. Apologising or briefly explaining to your patients why you are late as soon as they enter your room also often prevents them from venting their frustration.

Ask patients how much time they feel they need

A routine appointment of 10 minutes may be too long for a patient who just requires a signature, or too short for one who is presenting with serious problems. It may therefore be worth considering providing some flexibility for booking appointments, but you would need to check this out with your colleagues first. Many patients are very good at predicting the length of appointment that they require. When booking their slot, the receptionist could ask them how much time they think they will require, which may improve the flow of surgeries and help to reduce delays.

Restore your energy levels

Especially during long surgeries you may well become very hungry and thirsty, and the thought of missing your coffee or lunch break

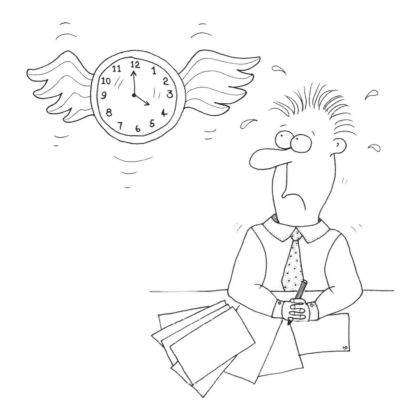

can be exasperating. For these 'dry spells' many GPs keep an emergency supply of fruit or other snacks and something to drink in their rooms, which helps them to maintain their stamina until the last patient has left. If you personally prefer chocolate, be aware that this may attract unwanted attention and should be kept in a safe place!

Take short breaks after difficult consultations

Seeing some of the more challenging patients can be very demanding and often requires considerable concentration and energy – it may even make you angry. If you feel exhausted after an arduous consultation, you could nip out through the back door and walk briskly round the surgery grounds. This only takes a couple of minutes, but can be very effective in restoring concentration and putting things back into perspective before you see your next patient.

Implementing change

Learning to manage change

Being unhappy about how your practice runs, or how the workload is distributed, may sometimes give rise to stress. Managing and introducing change are therefore important skills for GPs to develop, and there is no reason why this should not start at registrar level. However, no practice is perfect, and there is almost always more than one way of doing things, so before launching an attack on the current system it is usually a good idea to reflect on the history of your particular practice, and to find out whether any team members have a special fondness for the present way of working.

Strategies for implementing change

There are various reasons why change may be introduced in general practice. For example, change could be planned after discussion at a practice meeting, but it is sometimes imposed by the government or health authority, or can result from a serious incident that has happened in the practice. Change may also be the result of a personal idea suggested by a member of the practice team. This can be one way to help shape the way in which the practice runs or how the registrar training is conducted. In most cases it is best not to try to change everything at once. However, at the same time it is still important to try to keep alive the ideas and enthusiasm that people bring with them. Many experienced and successful GPs have developed strategies for getting things changed without upsetting everyone, and for making the change 'stick'. You can often learn a lot merely by observing your colleagues when they propose changes in practice meetings. For example, you can improve the chances of convincing your colleagues if you prepare photocopies of a short summary of what you would hope to achieve and the reasons why such a change may be beneficial. The outline could include a short background and the details and aims of the proposed modification, and could be backed up by recent relevant references from the literature, which would give such a proposal much more validity. It is important not to get too disheartened if, as happens in many cases, you meet with some degree of resistance from other team members – this is almost invariable and is part of the game. In the case of minor or less important issues, it may be as well to admit defeat early on and keep the peace rather than being too obstinate. However, if you feel very strongly about something there is no harm in persevering a little longer.

Stimulating others to come up with new ideas

Some practices work very well because they encourage all members of the team to make suggestions that save time, effort or money. For example, receptionists or practice nurses, who are experts in their fields, can often come up with the most ingenious proposals and ideas about how to make both their work and yours more effective. Why not suggest at one of the practice meetings that everyone tries to promote an atmosphere of striving for continuous improvement? For example, the team could ask everyone to provide at least one suggestion per meeting which could change their work or yours for the better. Another simple and often very productive method is to offer special incentives (a bottle of wine, gift voucher, etc.) for anyone in the practice who can come up with an idea that leads to significant improvements in practice organisation.

6 Jumping the hurdles: passing summative assessment and the MRCGP

Initial preparation

Summative assessment

Passing the MRCGP

The general practice registrar year has become busier in recent times. Passing summative assessment is now a requirement for becoming a fully qualified general practitioner, and you need to produce an audit project, prepare a video, sit a multiple-choice test and obtain a satisfactory trainer's report. Some registrars also decide to sit the MRCGP examination as well at the end of the registrar year, which may put an additional strain on them for a number of months. However, this is not as bad as it sounds. Most registrars manage all of this and still have time to enjoy themselves, although to be able to juggle all of the different assessments, it is very important to plan the year ahead. Try and sit down with your trainer early on and look at the official deadlines for the various assessments. For example, instead of leaving everything until the end, you may try to finish assignments such as the summative assessment multiple-choice question (MCQ) paper or the audit project at an early stage in order to leave more time for the video. By setting some personal deadlines, you may feel more in control, which can help you to monitor whether everything is running according to plan. However, this chapter is not intended to be a comprehensive guide to any of the examinations, but rather it attempts to look at some problem areas that may be worth considering.

Initial preparation

Getting essential papers signed

To be able to practise as a GP, you need to obtain a certificate of 'prescribed experience' after completion of the registrar year from the Joint Committee on Postgraduate Training for General Practice (JCPTGP), which is the statutory independent body that regulates training for general practice. You will be required to submit forms VTR 1 and 2 (available from your postgraduate department of general practice or from the regional adviser's office) for your registrar post and each hospital post counting towards your vocational training. Always confirm with the JCPTGP beforehand if you are uncertain whether your posts are accredited for general practice training. It is usually best to try to get these forms signed by your supervising hospital consultants immediately after each job, as there may be a delay in issuing your JCPTGP certificate if you leave it until the last minute. The forms can usually be submitted one month before the end of your training, or after completion of your registrar year.

Other practical assessments

Currently you will need to provide evidence of the ability to perform child health surveillance (including developmental assessment) and basic life support before you can sit the MRCGP. The relevant forms will be sent to you when you order the application pack, and you can be assessed by a health visitor and a hospital resuscitation officer or anaesthetist, respectively. It may take some time to sort out all of these matters and to arrange mutually convenient times, so the sooner you can obtain these certificates the better.

Learning about general practice

For many hospital jobs at SHO level it is often sufficient to read a short or medium-length textbook for that particular specialty (in addition to the formal teaching). However, learning about general practice is unique in many ways, as no single textbook can comprehensively cover all aspects of modern general practice. For this tremendously wide area you will need to be able to amalgamate facts yourself from a variety of different sources. Many past registrars would advise that you start reading around topics right from the beginning of the registrar year. However, time can often be at a premium, and because a vast amount of information is available, it is very easy to get sidetracked and lost in a wealth of detail. The most effective approach is often to obtain an overview of any new topic in the quickest way possible by reading only short summaries or reviews initially. Concentrating on the essential core facts first, and subsequently developing a broader knowledge base by filling in more detailed facts over the following months can be more productive than wading through large tomes which often contain much 'dead wood' in terms of their relevance to general practice. Try to become even more selective in what you read, and only look at papers and book sections that are relevant.

Summative assessment

Summative assessment has recently been introduced to provide evidence of GP registrars reaching a minimum acceptable standard before being allowed to work as independent general practitioners. Passing all four components is mandatory and should not prove too difficult for the majority of candidates. It should therefore be the aim to jump through these additional hoops as quickly as possible with minimal extra effort. Most Regional Offices for Summative Assessment organise courses about the various assessments which are well worth attending to give you an up-to-date overview. As the format may change from time to time, make sure that you always obtain the most recent instruction booklets.

Sit the MCQ examination on the first possible occasion

There is no harm in trying to sit this paper at a fairly early stage, as you may make multiple attempts. Even though some of the questions may appear rather difficult, most people pass first time. If you do fail, you will have gained some idea of the format and the areas on which you may need to concentrate, and if you pass first time, there is one less thing to worry about. General reading and study of review articles on major topics should be sufficient, and most candidates will require no special preparation.

Complete the audit project

Many registrars dread the thought of carrying out an audit project for summative assessment that may potentially be difficult and time-consuming. However, performing audits has become an integral part of general practice, and can actually be very interesting and stimulating. The key is to keep it as simple as possible, and to do it quickly. This reflects one of the aims of audit in terms of trying to improve your daily practice under time constraints. You may actually enjoy your project most if you concentrate on a small area and confine your audit to a single question. Many problems in general practice are complex, and these are often the ones that spring to mind first for an audit project. However, for the purpose of summative assessment it is important to force yourself to find a very simple question that interests you, and to concentrate on that question alone. Always remember that this is not a PhD thesis but only an exercise in showing that you have grasped the essentials of the audit process.

Choose a topic for which data are already available

Much time can potentially be spent on collecting data for your project. For this reason it may be an advantage to select an audit that uses data which are already available in the practice, such as laboratory results or appointment bookings. You can then start to process case-notes or other data immediately and get on with the project without having to wait for data to be generated.

Select a problem for which routine practice can be improved

One of the most important issues to consider is whether your audit provides the potential for change. Looked at from this angle, many potential questions involving the quality of care will become obvious. Potential projects may include the mentioning of essential facts in referral letters or the prescription of recommended drugs for certain conditions, but almost any area can be chosen for an audit. A new and innovative audit is much more interesting to carry out, and may even be more likely to pass.

Set yourself a deadline for completion of the audit project

Even if you seem to have plenty of time on your hands at the beginning of the year, the months do pass very quickly. For this reason you may want to try to get the audit out of the way early on, and it can help if you set yourself a deadline. A simple audit should probably not take much longer than 8–12 hours at the most, including research, data collection and writing up. If it takes longer, your question may be too complicated or difficult. Discuss your audit plan with your trainer and peers, who may be very helpful in narrowing the question down.

Write up your audit as you go along

Even during the research phase, think of the audit report that you will need to submit. Some GPs would suggest writing down all of the points or arguments you would like to mention in the report under their respective headings (e.g. reasons for choosing the audit, criteria, recommendations, etc.), preferably on index cards. Whenever you have a new idea that you would like to include, you can write it on a new card and add it to the others. You can then easily put the cards in order under their headings. Writing up will be more straightforward, as you will only need to concentrate on one point at a time.

Prepare the video

Two areas that commonly cause problems during the making of the video for summative assessment or the MRCGP are technical hiccups and general logistics. It does not take very long to get used to seeing yourself on camera, but sorting out technical faults can take a while and may become frustrating. This may lead to potentially very good consultations being scrapped for reasons such as insufficient light or poor sound. Getting the set-up right from the start can help to reduce hours of re-recording and editing. Many video cameras can seem to have a personality of their own and need to be handled in a certain way. Technophobes in particular should get hold of the manual and read the relevant sections before starting to record. Knowing exactly what every button does and how to operate the camera is essential for obtaining a satisfactory result. You may also find that your machine is able to show the time and date on the recording, which is a definite advantage. With time you will gain increasing confidence and feel much more at ease using the machine.

Perform trial runs with a friend or your trainer

Your video may be rejected for reasons of poor technical quality, so it is essential to try to produce high-quality recordings. Consulting rooms vary in size and shape, and it is advisable to try to create the best possible recording conditions, which usually involves some experimenting with sound, light, camera position and room layout. Using a colleague, friend or your trainer as a 'dummy patient' to experiment with different camera settings can help you to get things right from the start, without the additional stresses that are present during consultations. For recordings to be accepted, it is necessary to show the faces of both the doctor and the patient. To achieve this you may need to try out various camera positions and rearrange your room if necessary. Find a secure position for the camera where it cannot be knocked over or moved accidentally. This is important for safety reasons, and it also reduces the risk of your videos suddenly showing only your feet after someone has accidentally bumped into the stand. Many cameras do not function very well in direct light, so you may want to try to record away from any windows. Alternatively, you could draw the curtains and use artificial light, rather than risk poor picture quality.

Aim for good sound quality

Examiners are often unable to follow consultations due to poor sound quality, which in many cases could have been avoided. Some video cameras have built-in microphones that only work well if the subjects are very close and in line with the microphone. In many situations, an external microphone can dramatically improve results, but it needs to be carefully placed. If it is placed directly on the desk, even writing or putting your stethoscope down can cause irritating background noise. If your printer is rather loud, consider writing prescriptions by hand when using the video.

Book special 'video surgeries'

The video for summative assessment only requires a routine case-mix that represents typical 'bread-and-butter' general practice problems. You may therefore be able to submit a complete surgery without having to go to all the trouble of editing your tape. For this reason, ask your receptionists to book a whole surgery as a 'video surgery', and then you will not have to arrange and switch on the video for individual patients, but can leave it running for the entire session. It is also worth considering making these video appointments slightly longer in order to cater for any delays in connection with the recording.

Increase the consent rate for your video sessions

Every patient needs to sign a consent form. Some only refuse to be filmed because they would have combed their hair specially or worn different clothes if they had known in advance that they were going to be taped. Therefore you should explain carefully to your receptionists exactly what the video is for. This is important, as a positive attitude among the receptionists towards videos is more likely to be passed on to your patients. The receptionists can inform patients as soon as they book an appointment that in this particular surgery they will be filmed, and that anyone who does not wish to give their consent will be allocated an alternative slot. When the patients turn up for their appointments, the receptionists can then hand out the consent forms for them to sign. You will merely have to collect the forms as each patient enters your room, thus avoiding much of the bureaucracy. Consent forms need to be signed again by the patient at the end of the consultation, and you can put an *aide-mémoire* on your desk or the inside of your door to remind yourself about this. However, if you forget you can usually obtain the signature retrospectively by sending the consent form to the patient for signing, together with a stamped addressed envelope.

Don't leave the video until the last minute

Many registrars shy away from being video-taped out of fear of not recording a 'perfect' consultation. However, viewed realistically, it would be almost impossible to find even experienced GPs who always consult faultlessly, so don't become obsessive, but rather try to produce some trial videos early in the registrar year so that you get used to being video-taped. Try to recognise any major areas of weakness that you can work on over the following months. Do not worry too much if you find your first attempts excruciating – everyone goes through this phase and feels the same. This is also a very valuable exercise for improving your consultation technique, and will probably be part of your training in any case. Practice is certainly one of the keys.

Get feedback on the final video tape

The main aim of summative assessment is to show that you are a safe doctor and know your limitations. If you are aware of any shortcomings in your recorded consultations, make sure that you mention them in the log-book to show that you are conscious of them. However, it is very important to view the tape with your trainer in order to be absolutely sure you have not made any major mistakes that may fail you. Although most people feel embarrassed when viewing recordings of themselves with someone else present, it is essential to obtain feedback in order to avoid sending in a tape of dubious standard.

Look at the trainer's report with your trainer

Rather than leaving the trainer's report until the end of the training, most of the items can be filled in during the year as you progress. Go through the form with your trainer, and make a list of procedures that need to be observed. For example, if you know how to perform a cervical smear and feel confident enough to do it correctly, ask your trainer to watch you during the procedure, so he or she can fill in the trainer's report subsequently. If your technique needs improvement, this would probably be a good time to obtain feedback. Another useful opportunity for starting to complete the trainer's report is during joint consultations with your trainer.

Passing the MRCGP

The MRCGP examination aims to test skills and knowledge to a higher degree than summative assessment, and requires slightly different examination preparation. The areas tested tend to be much wider, and include topics such as ethics, practice management, research, clinical topics and new developments in primary care. You will probably need to start planning your preparation early in the registrar year if you decide to sit this examination, as there is a considerable amount of reading involved. One advantage of attempting the examination during the registrar year is that taking part in the day-release course already covers wide areas of your preparation. If you pass first time, you will be able to relax after the year, and may have an advantage when applying for jobs. It is probably also easier to form a study group during the registrar year. However, you will need to invest a fair amount of time and effort, and you may feel slightly pressured. If you are unsure whether to prepare for this examination at this stage, talk to your friends, colleagues and trainer, and perhaps consider attempting only one or two of the four modules initially. Again, although the amount of preparation required can seem substantial, most registrars still manage to really enjoy their registrar year and have enough time left for other interests.

The examination itself

The format of the MRCGP examination has developed and changed over the past few years. At present the examination is modular, which means that you can sit each of the four components (MCQ, modified essay questions (MEQ), video and oral examination) individually. It is quite a relief not to have to resit the whole examination if you fail one or more modules. The examination format is also sometimes subject to change, and it is therefore essential to have a detailed knowledge of the examination requirements and to obtain the latest examination regulations from the Royal College of General Practitioners before starting your revision. These regulations also contain much useful advice and are worth looking at carefully. You should also obtain an up-to-date book on examination technique, and use every opportunity to ask previous candidates about their experiences with summative assessment and the MRCGP. With their help and by reading the leader articles in the *British Medical Journal, British Journal of General Practice* and the free medico-political publications it will be much easier to draw up a list of 'hot topics' that can guide and focus your preparation. Other useful sources of information include articles about examination technique in the medico-political magazines, which are often written by MRCGP examiners. The Royal College, some regional GP postgraduate departments and a number of commercial companies also offer revision courses that may be worth attending, and you can often obtain information about their quality from previous registrars.

Joining or starting a study group

Learning about general practice and preparing for the examination is far more effective in a group than on your own – in addition to generally being much more fun. One of the main advantages is that much of the work can be shared. It is also much easier to cope with difficult periods when spirits are low, as moral support is so important during the months of revision. Some groups find it useful to meet in each member's home on a rotating basis and have dinner together. There are various ways in which different aspects of the examination can be tackled. Many study groups decide to distribute a number of topics to each group member at the beginning, and then fill in a diary for the next two to four months, stating who is to do some research and present summaries of certain topics on a particular date. This way you will know in advance when it is your turn to prepare a topic, and it may also be much easier to judge whether all of the relevant subjects can be covered in the given time. You may also do critical reading exercises together, or brainstorm ideas for answering the MEQ paper. Study group sessions should be enjoyable, but if there are serious personality clashes in your group that cannot be resolved amicably, it may be best to change groups early on.

Keeping a file with references and summaries of hot topics

Collecting relevant information in conjunction with examination preparation is a time-consuming business and can be very tedious. For this reason, try to get in touch with previous registrars who have sat the MRCGP, or your postgraduate centre, and obtain copies of important references, or even complete study folders which only need to be updated. It is often best to collect copies of landmark papers, relevant systematic reviews and national guidelines, and to file them alphabetically according to topic. If you start such a file for your training practice as well, this can be of value to future registrars, and it can also be updated by any other partners in the practice who come across relevant or important material.

Using index cards

In the run-up to the examinations it is often impossible to wade through all of the papers that you have accumulated over the preceding months. It is therefore sometimes useful to write summaries of most topics on index cards. If you try to condense each topic or subtopic on to one card, you will be forced to be concise and to the point.

Preparing for the MCQ paper

In most instances general reading and studying the hot topics that you have defined in your study group will form the basis for passing the MCQ paper. It is important to be aware of review articles and editorials on important topics in the *British Medical Journal* and *British Journal of General Practice* over at least the preceding couple of years. Many of the political issues relevant to general practice are discussed in the free GP papers, and these articles give you a fairly good idea of current hot topics. Try to obtain sample questions (the free journals regularly contain pages with practice MCQs) and revise your areas of weakness by reading short textbooks for the respective specialties, rather than tackling every specialty in detail. When you order the application form from the college you will also receive an information booklet which contains the current outline and format of the questions.

Critical appraisal skills

Critical appraisal of the medical literature in the light of evidence-based medicine has become an integral part of the MRCGP examination, and questions on this topic may appear in the MCQ paper or in other parts of the examination, including the viva. Because keeping up to date in the field of general practice requires extensive reading, it is helpful to develop techniques for summarising the evidence in order to avoid information overload. It can be very time-consuming to revise all of the journals during the weeks before the examination, and reducing the information to bite-size chunks can help dramatically. To aid your revision, you may consider writing the essentials of relevant papers on index cards and highlighting the core features whenever you read a paper or editorial that is relevant. However, try not to get bogged down in too much detail, as it is really far more important to remember the main points of many key papers than to be able to recall the intricate details of just a few. It takes some time to get used to reading original research papers critically, but with time and practice you will find that it becomes much easier to assess articles fairly quickly.

Getting a feel for important current issues

If you have time, it is advisable to go through recent issues of the *British Medical Journal* and the *British Journal of General Practice* in more detail. However, if you only have a few days left before the examination, even skimming through the editorials and the summary page will give you a rough idea of which topics are currently under debate. You can now also find a lot of useful information on the Internet. Try to think of the strengths and

Table 6.1 Points to consider when critically appraising a paper

1 General comments
- Reputable source (authors, journal, sponsorship)?
- Helpful layout?

2 Title and summary
- Subject relevant to own practice?
- Does it tackle a clearly answerable question?
- Conclusion applicable ('generalisable') to practice population?

3 Introduction
- Identifying gaps of knowledge?
- Adequate literature search?

4 Methods/study design
- Clear statement of the purpose of the study? Clear outcome measurements?
- Study design (observational/ interventional, prospective/ retrospective, blinding, randomisation)?
- Participants (How randomised? Similar to practice population? When, where and how recruited? Sample size large enough? Control group adequate and similar to intervention group? Inclusion/ exclusion criteria reasonable?)
- Interventions (Clearly stated? Control intervention defined?)
- Outcome measurement (Objective measurements used? How measured? *If a questionnaire*: structure, validity, reliability? Response rate? Non-responders examined? Questions unbiased? *If an intervention*: follow-up length? Drop-outs accounted for? Side effects sought? All relevant information obtained?

5 Results
- Clearly stated and presented? Do figures and text match? All participants accounted for? Losses to follow-up and drop-outs analysed? Expressed in useful ways (absolute risk reduction (ARR), odds ratio (OR), number needed to treat (NNT))? Analysis on 'intention-to-treat' basis? How large was treatment effect? Fully analysed? Do results fulfil aims of the study? 'Net impact' of the study? Confidence limits given?

6 Discussion/conclusions
- Clearly stated? Any conclusions not supported by facts? Alternative explanations discussed? Relevant to your patients? Implications for healthcare?
- Recommendations justified? Cost-effectiveness? Need for further research discussed? References up to date and relevant? Should findings be acted upon?

weaknesses of each argument, and attempt to form your own opinion on every topic.

Tackling the MEQ paper

This paper assesses, among other things, whether you are able to consider all of the important issues in conjunction with, for example, a clinical case scenario, an ethical dilemma or a new development in general practice. As you will not be marked for style, you can increase your score by developing an effective way of presenting as much information as possible within the limited time available. Answering this type of question takes a little practice. Try

---

Table 6.2 Examples of points to consider when answering modified essay questions

1 Patient
- Hidden agenda
- Underlying physical, psychological and social problems
- Autonomy and rights
- Confidentiality
- Factors influencing adherence to treatment
- Why presenting now?
- Present coping strategies
- Patient's point of view
- Health beliefs
- Non-verbal clues
- Abuse/family or child at risk
- HIV risk

2 Doctor
- Implications (time, workload, financial, future care, medico-legal aspects, etc.)
- Effect on subsequent consultations
- Appreciate limitations within single consultation
- Ethical dilemmas
- Own feelings (guilt, anger, blame)
- Prescribing problems
- Emotional content
- Establishing rapport
- Exploring patient's wishes
- Discovering connections between presentations
- Information gathering and obtaining baseline data
- Management plan (e.g. history, examination, investigations, referral)
- Discussion with and involvement of primary healthcare team

- Stress (appreciate normal emotions, be aware of emotional turmoil, postponing on-call or major decisions, etc.)
- Provide information (be aware of principles: small amounts, non-technical language, simplicity, check understanding, opportunity for questions)
- Show empathy and appreciate problems
- Review medication and current symptoms
- Breaking bad news (language, content, pace of information giving, setting, relatives, what they have been told so far, check understanding, offer contact and help)

3 Others
- Patient's family and friends (appreciate role of family as unit)
- Multidisciplinary approach in primary healthcare team (including receptionist, nurse, occupational therapist, physiotherapist, special community services, etc.)
- Hospital specialists
- Society as a whole
- Neighbours

4 General
- Advantages and drawbacks
- Risks and benefits
- Security for staff and yourself

to obtain old examination questions or think up your own, and in your study group ask everyone to come up with as many different angles to a problem as possible. After a while you will feel much more confident about answering this type of question, and it will also be of great benefit for your daily practice, as you will get used to looking at problems from every possible viewpoint.

Structuring your answers

The examiners will mark your paper with the help of a marking grid containing constructs, which are a type of model answer that a group of examiners consider to contain the most important aspects of a particular topic. Most good answers would require you to cover four or five main aspects of a problem in sufficient detail. You will get higher marks by covering all aspects reasonably well than if you only deal with one or two in great detail, so you need to structure your answer. For example, you may start by dividing the answer page into different headings. For a clinical scenario these could include, say, history, examination, hidden agenda, ethical considerations, doctor's own feelings, confidentiality or other headings, depending on the problem. You will only have 10 to 15 minutes per question, and it is much easier to get higher marks by using bullet points and providing lists. This also makes marking less tedious for the examiners. Start off broadly by filling in the space below your headings, and gradually provide more and more detail until you have reached the limits of your knowledge or the end of the 10 minutes available. In the run-up to the examination you may want to make a list of points to consider, and read briefly through the list every day. This will help you to have the main issues at your fingertips and to tailor them to specific questions. The Royal College of General Practitioners application pack also includes a list of areas of competence that will be tested in the examination.

Polishing your video

In contrast to the video recording required for summative assessment, you are encouraged to edit the video for the MRCGP and to submit a variety of consultations that show you in your best light. Make sure that you leave plenty of time for editing the final tape, as this will often take far longer than you expect. The instruction booklet for the video recording is very open about the marking criteria. Try to mark some of your own video consultations together with your trainer, or in your study group, against those criteria. If you continually fall short in a particular area, you could place a list of these criteria in front of you on your desk or wall as a reminder, and ask yourself after each consultation whether you have covered everything. You will soon notice any regular omissions, and can then concentrate on including these in future consultations.

Approaching the oral examination

Oral examinations can generate considerable anxiety in many candidates, who often find it difficult to prepare for this part of the examination. However, studying viva technique and psychological preparation are probably as important as revising the important topics in general practice. In the weeks before the viva, it can help to get used to the sound of your own voice by regularly reading aloud, or practising answers by talking to yourself, perhaps in front of a mirror. As many questions are very open, you may want to prepare yourself to be able to talk for at least a couple of minutes on a particular topic, and develop structures for answering different types of questions. Some of these may involve a case scenario and end with the question 'What would you do?', while others could ask your opinion on a particular topic, such as 'What do you think about research in general practice?' or 'What is your opinion on genetically modified food?'. Instead of immediately expressing your own thoughts, it is often much better to give an outline of the debate, and only then to present your own view on the matter. Include in your answers the advantages and disadvantages or costs and benefits of any problematic topic, to show that you have considered both sides of the argument before presenting (and perhaps defending) your own opinion.

Preparing some standard sentences to cool your nerves

Often the most difficult part of answering a question is getting started. Some questions can be answered with initial standard sentences and phrases that may give you a few seconds to structure your reply. For instance, you could summarise a problem by saying 'I think the issue in this case scenario is (break of confidentiality, a hidden agenda, illegal prescribing, etc.)', giving the examiner a chance to interrupt should you be missing the point before you embark on a lengthy discussion of the topic. If you start your answer with a phrase such as 'I think this question raises the following issues: 1. . ., 2. . ., 3. . .', you can outline your answer first and then deal with each point in turn, having already demonstrated that you have a plan for your reply. Even if you do not get time to finish your answer, the examiners will then know that you have thought of the remaining areas as well.

Practising answering under pressure

Together with your study group, try to arrange a mock viva with someone who is or was an MRCGP examiner, such as a local trainer or your course organiser. This can be invaluable, as it will put you on the spot and give you some idea of what the viva may be like. However, do not be disheartened if the mock examination is stressful and does not go well – the real examination is often much easier to cope with!

Preparing yourself psychologically

Certain behaviour of the examiners may be unexpected, and it can be helpful to anticipate some of their reactions. Most examiners will be very friendly, but the atmosphere may be rather business-like, as they will concentrate on asking questions and marking your answers. Do not expect much feedback on your performance, and concentrate on the next question even if you feel that you have performed poorly in a previous answer, because all of the questions will be marked independently. Oral examinations are always to some extent an artificial situation, and it is natural to become nervous in this setting. When facing the examiners, you could try to imagine yourself leading a slightly difficult consultation with one of your patients and a relative (a situation which by now you can probably handle very well, and which you are much more used to). Finally, remember that examiners want to stretch you to the limit, so if the going gets tough and the questions become more difficult, you are likely to be doing very well. Good luck!

7 Ready for take-off: flying solo as a new general practitioner

Working as a locum

Joining a partnership

Dipping into other ponds

A variety of job options are available to GP registrars on completion of their training. Starting as a GP locum is probably one of the most popular choices straight after the registrar year, as it allows new GPs to be flexible and provides the opportunity to work in many different practices before settling into a more permanent position – if they wish to do so. There are many other exciting areas in which you can work as a GP if you do not want to become a principal in general practice straight away. This chapter looks briefly at locum work and becoming a principal, and ends with a short summary of other options.

Working as a locum

Obtain up-to-date information about your rights and responsibilities

Becoming a locum involves a change to being self-employed, which basically requires you to set up your own business. You will commonly be working in different practices, and this can have the advantage of providing experience of a variety of working environments (you may even find your future practice among one of these). It also means becoming responsible for your own financial affairs and having the freedom to determine your personal working pattern. The local Department of Social Security (DSS) provides free leaflets that contain some useful general information about issues to consider when becoming self-employed. Your national insurance (NI) contributions are normally deducted from your salary if you are employed, but as a locum you need to pay NI contributions yourself, so contact your local NI office to arrange payments. Unfortunately, benefits such as sick pay and paid holidays are lost, and it is currently under debate whether you will be able to make contributions to the NHS superannuation scheme in the future.

Have all of the obligatory papers available

It is vital that you can prove to the practices that you fulfil all of the necessary formal requirements for being employed as a locum. For your own protection, it is essential that your medical indemnity subscription is valid and up to date. Although the subscription is costly, it can often be paid in instalments. If you only work part-time, you may be eligible for a reduced rate, and it is worth enquiring about this. Make sure that your General Medical Council (GMC) certificate is valid and have copies ready to send out with your applications. You should also be able to provide copies of the Certificate of Prescribed Experience issued by the JCPTGP.

Contact local non-principal groups and national organisations

Working on your own can be quite lonely and difficult initially, especially if you had a very supportive trainer and training practice. Therefore it is important to try to keep in touch with your old practice and with other ex-trainees, even if you move. You should definitely consider joining your local non-principal group, which is headed by the National Association of Non-Principals (NANP). This relatively young organisation represents non-principals nationwide and provides information and advice on matters concerning general practice. The NANP also represents the interests of non-principals and aims to improve their working conditions. Information is published in a newsletter, by emails to members, on a web site, and in an excellent handbook full of practical information and useful tips. Most local non-principal groups meet regularly about once a month and provide an opportunity to exchange views about issues concerning, for example, locum work and information about local practices, as well as news on continuing medical education. They will help you to assess your own expectations and experiences and to compare them with those of your peers. These meetings are also a very good source of mutual support and tend to be very sociable occasions which help you to get to know people if you are new to an area. The local BMA office may also be able to advise on local pay rates, and can give advice on a variety of other matters concerning locums.

Replenish stocks in your doctor's bag

You will be able to obtain drugs for your bag from your local pharmacist by private prescription. Many pharmacists are very helpful and can give good advice on cheaper options, and may even offer discounts. Type a list of drugs that you require with your name, address and GMC number at the top. Specify that the drugs are for your bag, and sign and date the list at the bottom. Some parenteral drugs are only available in larger packets, and you may want to share vials among a group of locums. Always keep receipts for tax purposes, as all purchases of medical equipment and drugs count as business expenses and are tax deductible. Buy a notebook in which to keep a permanent record of controlled drugs that you carry and supply. If you do little out-of-hours work and have access to drugs supplied by, for instance, a co-operative, a full drugs supply in your bag is probably unnecessary. However, it is essential to keep a basic stock of emergency drugs.

Decide what kind of work you would like to do

There are many different ways of working as a locum, and each has its advantages and disadvantages. You may want to look for a potential practice to join as a principal, in which case it would be a good idea to work in a variety of practices to see what they are like. However, this way of working can become rather disruptive after a while, and if you already have a job lined up for the future and would prefer a stable position with regular hours of work, it may be more appropriate to look for relatively long-term posts such as maternity or sabbatical locums, although these may give you less flexibility. Some practices employ locums because a partner has left, and working there may be a good opportunity to get to know the other partners. If you are planning to continue working straight after completing your training, it is advisable to start looking for work a few months ahead, as it always takes some time for jobs to come up. Locum work usually gives you a certain amount of flexibility, so this may be a good opportunity to develop new skills and take up regular sessions in areas that interest you, such as family planning or sessions in a prison.

Get yourself known in the area

Deputising services and locum agencies often try to recruit locums through advertisements in the medical press. However, many locums look for suitable practices themselves and bypass the agencies. You can find practice addresses and telephone numbers in the yellow pages, or by requesting a list from the local health authority. This will enable you to do a mailshot of all the practices that regularly need locums. Most health authorities also have a locum list on which you can ask to be included. Contact your local postgraduate department and let them know that you are available for work, as they are often asked about new locums in the area. It is usually a good policy to try to visit practices in which you would like to work and to meet the practice manager in person. Telephone the practices regularly and ask whether work is coming up. You can also write postcards to the practice manager as a reminder that you are still available. Do not be put off if work only comes in slowly at the beginning. Persistence often pays, as there is a very high rate of turnover. Although initially you will be applying to the practice, in many cases the secretaries or receptionists are the ones who will be asked to contact locums. For this reason, you may want to get some small business cards printed (this can be done fairly cheaply in copy shops or by automatic machines in shopping centres) containing all of the necessary details. Include a couple of these with your application, so that they can be pinned up on the office notice-board, where your details will be much more readily available than in a CV that is filed away in a folder.

Make it easy for practices to contact you

Most practices will try to contact you during working hours, so it is important that they can get hold of you easily, or leave a message if you are working elsewhere. This is especially important for any last-minute bookings. An answerphone is probably the minimum requirement, and it should have a facility to allow you to check messages by phone from elsewhere. Your message on the machine should ask practices to leave an evening telephone number or a fax number which you can contact. It may also be worth investing in a pager or mobile phone. A pager has the advantage that you can phone back in your own time and do not have to negotiate locum work in the middle of a consultation. Try to obtain one that has a vibration function to avoid unnecessary interruption. A fax machine is a more costly but very helpful addition, as you can respond to any messages outside working hours. It is very easy to confuse times and dates when accepting locum work, so try at all costs to avoid double-bookings or forgetting sessions that you have accepted. For this reason, too, it is a good idea to get a wall planner in addition to your diary, and make sure that you update both regularly.

Table 7.1 Points to consider when applying for locum posts	
• Length of surgeries and number of appointments	• Daytime on-call
• Consultation rate	• Out-of-hours
• Extra patients	• Visits
• Paperwork (including prescriptions)	• Emergencies
• Nurse available?	• Locum pack available?

Negotiate your rates

There are no fixed rates for locum pay, which may vary between practices and depend on location, locum availability and season. The BMA provides recommendations for locum rates, but these are only suggestions that form a basis for negotiations. Find out from other locums in the area what the current rates are, and negotiate rates with the practices, which should be confirmed in writing. It is often useful to find out in advance what is expected from you. For instance, you may be happy to accept slightly lower rates for a very relaxed surgery with long appointments. Generally speaking, the longer the period of work, the more you need to know about the practice and your work commitments. It is important that both you and the practice have a similar idea of your workload, and the details should be confirmed in writing. Most practices have different ways of paying, so you need to have a reliable method of keeping an overview of your invoices and any payments received. If you do not get paid on the day, send an invoice immediately and ask to be paid within one week. You can buy invoice books that print through a copy for you to keep whenever you issue an invoice. When you receive payments, record any details against the entries in your diary or on your wall planner, where it will be easy to keep track of your finances. Another approach is to record all payment details in separate files for both paid and unpaid salaries, which should give you a good overview of which practices have paid and which have not.

Use a spreadsheet for outgoing expenses

A useful method for keeping track of expenses is to have a simple spreadsheet (preferably on a computer program) for each month, in which you enter details of payments, transport, professional subscriptions, stationery, telephone expenses and other outgoings. Update your records regularly to avoid the need to backtrack any expenses. Make sure that you keep all relevant receipts in a safe place, as you may need these at a later stage for tax purposes. Remember that you can claim back tax on all legitimate business expenses such as mileage for work, costs of running an 'office' in your home, professional fees and pensions. Therefore as well as keeping mileage records and writing down all expenses related to your car ownership, you should also keep a record of your personal car mileage. You will be able to claim a proportion of the cost of your heating and electricity if you use an area of your home for work, and you can claim for business phone use as well. A free leaflet, available from the tax office, provides more details about the expenses that are tax deductible. To avoid running into debt when you face the inevitable tax bill, you may want to pay 25 to 30% of your gross earnings immediately into a separate account. This should amply cover the tax bill, and will probably also provide a small bonus for you at the end of the tax year.

Get help from an accountant

The costs involved in employing an accountant depend on the extent to which they need to sort out your financial affairs. Ideally you will have prepared your accounts yourself, and they should only need to approve. To find an accountant, you could ask your training practice about their accountant or speak to other locum colleagues. You can often negotiate a fee, and you should always ask for a written quote.

Look after yourself

As you are not entitled to sick pay as a locum, it is important to consider taking out personal health insurance and life cover, especially if you have any dependents. It is worth obtaining information about this and talking to an independent financial adviser. Also try to pencil in some holidays for yourself, as it is very easy to find yourself accepting more and more work once the ball is rolling. Unfortunately, you will not get any 'paid' leave, but if you recharge your batteries every so often, your work as a locum will be much more efficient and enjoyable.

Support the practices in which you work

Locums form an integral part of modern general practice, and their work is essential for the running of many GP surgeries. To become even better recognised as a professional group, it is important that locums try to integrate themselves into practices as much as possible. It can make life much easier for the employing principals if you manage patients as if you were their own GP. This also avoids creating the impression that locums only deal with simple and straightforward problems.

Joining a partnership

Outline your ideal practice before you apply

When looking for a practice that you would like to join as a principal, the variety that is available can be overwhelming. It can be useful to write down all the desired features of your ideal practice, not that you are likely to find your ideal post easily, but you may come very close if you decide on your preferences in advance. For instance, the practice area can greatly influence the type of work you will be doing. There is a huge difference between rural and inner-city practices, and even within those areas the demographic features may vary and can have a significant impact on your work. If you plan to live near your practice, you may want to consider your personal needs and those of your family. Factors such as house prices, public transport, and the availability of nurseries, schools and leisure facilities could play an important role in determining which practices you approach. Before applying for principal posts, it is often best to be clear in your own mind which features of a new job are important for you and your family and which are not. Do not go for posts that have any features which would be unacceptable to you.

Consider your optimum workload

Your working pattern will largely depend on the general attitude of the principals. If you prefer to have longer appointments, shorter surgeries, more time off and a generally more relaxed working atmosphere, but are prepared to accept a lower income, you probably do not want to join 'workaholic' colleagues who may be high-earning but stretched to the limit. Your professional goals and aspirations are also worth bearing in mind. If you have any special interests that you wish to develop, it is important to know whether your future practice will be able to accommodate these. If you want to do research, you may want to be close to an academic department of general practice. If you plan to become a GP trainer in the future, in many cases it will be easier if you join an already established training practice rather than setting up everything yourself. If you have any special clinical interests and want to work as a clinical assistant, you will need to be fairly near a suitable hospital.

Update your CV

A good CV is the key to being short-listed for an interview. Using a decent word-processing package and laser printouts on good-quality paper will make a more favourable impression. Clear presentation and layout will make your CV easier to read, and may just tip the balance in your favour during the short-listing process. A considerable amount of detail should be included to help your potential employer to gain an initial impression of your background and assess your suitability as a future partner. Try to emphasise those areas of your experience that would be relevant for a particular practice setting.

Use the opportunity to interview your potential new partners

In most cases a general practice partnership is a long-term commitment, and both sides should make every effort to find out whether your appointment is likely to work in the long term. There are many reasons why a partnership may have come up. Retirement, partnership disagreements, partners going part-time or illness due to stress may all require a practice to look for a new principal. There is usually no harm in finding out why a practice wants to recruit a new partner. There may be certain qualities that they are looking for in their potential new colleague, which may already give you an indication as to whether that practice would be suitable for you. Decide what kind of working relationship you would like to have with your future colleagues, and try to find out about their philosophies, interests and general involvement in practice affairs. Consider whether you would be prepared to work in a slightly hierarchical structure, or whether you would prefer to be treated equally from the start. You also need to decide how important meeting the other partners on a regular basis is for you, as this can vary a lot from one practice to another.

Check the practice accounts and practice organisation

As you will be part of a business, it is important that you know whether your future practice is being managed well, and your earning prospects. As soon as both you and the practice have indicated that the job could be yours, ask whether you can look at the practice accounts, together with either your own or the practice accountant. Also look at the way in which additional income is distributed, as this can be shared or paid on an individual basis, which may be of major significance in certain circumstances. You need to know exactly how the practice property is owned before accepting a position as a principal, and whether it belongs to all of the partners. Other important features are the time you will need to reach financial parity, provision of out-of-hours care (whether it is provided by the practice or a co-operative/deputising service), daytime on-call (how it is organised and whether it is divided equally among the partners) and whether the practice has shared or personal lists. In a rural setting you may be required to provide intrapartum care or to look after GP beds in the local community hospital. You may also need to perform rather more minor surgery in a remote area if the nearest casualty department is some distance away. In addition, you need to consider how much you value good access to a district general hospital or teaching hospital with good specialist facilities.

The partnership agreement

Practice affairs can be handled in many different ways and are worth knowing about in advance. You should find out how holidays and study or sick leave are dealt with, and whether there is the possibility of taking sabbatical leave. Another important issue is the decision-making process (is there a right to veto any decision?). You need to know where the responsibilities for debts and tax lie, and whether there is an agreed procedure in disputes. The General Medical Services Council (GMSC) of the BMA provides guidance on partnership issues in the form of a free booklet which contains very useful advice and check-lists. Be very careful if a practice does not have a written partnership agreement, and be wary about accepting any post unless you have a written document outlining how potential areas of dispute would be dealt with.

Dipping into other ponds

A number of alternatives are available for newly qualified general practitioners who may find locum work too unsettling and a principal position within a partnership too permanent to start with. You may become involved in research, police or prison work, medical writing, expeditions or exchanges, teaching, medical politics or any of numerous other areas that interest you. Some of the more common and popular options are briefly mentioned below.

General practice assistantships

Many practices employ assistants who are fully qualified GPs but do not have the status of a partner. This may be a good option if you have other commitments such as childcare, or want to be able to leave a post quickly should you need to follow your partner to another area. You will have to deal with fewer administrative issues, but can enjoy continuity of care for your patients. You may also have fewer on-call commitments, and you will have rights within the employment law, including maternity pay and sick leave. You can obtain up-to-date information on issues concerning working contracts from the BMA.

Clinical assistants

Many GPs have special clinical interests and take up a part-time clinical assistantship at the local hospital. A half or full day a week in specialties such as dermatology, cardiology, accident and emergency or any other area can be of benefit both to yourself and to the practice in which you work. Many posts are short-term on a renewable basis and may be a good way to improve your skills and expertise in a particular field.

Retainees

The main aim of the retainer scheme is to keep GPs in touch with medical practice while they are taking a career break. You may find posts by approaching local postgraduate departments or contacting practices directly. Working as a retainee enables you to work for a limited number of sessions and to attend postgraduate teaching. You will be able to join the NHS pension scheme and can usually negotiate a contract with your employing practice. Practices participating in the retainer scheme need to be approved by the various regions and should reach the standard of a training practice.

Hospital posts

Many newly qualified GPs return to hospital to work for another six or 12 months as an SHO in a specialty in which they would like to gain more experience. Having worked in general practice may make it much easier to concentrate on learning the skills relevant for GPs, and subjects such as family planning, dermatology, ENT and ophthalmology are commonly chosen.

Academic general practice

The prospects for young GPs intending to enter a career in academic general practice have improved immensely recently. During the last few years more grants and support have been made available for primary care research. It is usually best to contact an academic department in your area to find out about the local options. You could, for example, be helping with an established research project initially, which would be a good way to find out whether you do like this kind of work. If you become seriously interested you may, together with the department, submit an application for a research training fellowship. This would usually last three years and includes both training and research components. These training grants are given out by the Wellcome

Foundation, the Medical Research Council and local or national NHS Research and Development funds, and would cover your training expenses plus a clinical salary. The Royal College of General Practitioners also offers similar types of research fellowships. Generally speaking, your salary would not be as high as that of a principal, but you will usually have less clinical responsibility and fewer on-call commitments, and will often be able to obtain a higher degree. Research is usually combined with sessions in general practice to keep up your clinical skills and allow you to develop new ideas for research questions.

Suggested reading

Consultation

Liversey PG (1996) *The GP Consultation. A Registrar's Guide* (2e). Butterworth-Heinemann, Oxford.

Neighbour R (1996) *The Inner Consultation*. Petroc Press, Newbury.

Pendleton D, Schofield T, Tate P and Havelock P (1984, reprinted 1997) *The Consultation*. Oxford General Practice Series. Oxford University Press, Oxford.

Tate P (1997) *The Doctor's Communication Handbook* (2e). Radcliffe Medical Press, Oxford.

MRCGP

Crombie I (1996) *The Pocket Guide to Critical Appraisal*. BMJ Publishing Group, London.

Ellis N (2000) *General Practitioner's Handbook* (2e). Radcliffe Medical Press, Oxford.

Greenhalgh T (1997) *How to Read a Paper. The Basics of Evidence-Based Medicine*. BMJ Publishing Group, London.

Palmer KT (1997) *Notes for the MRCGP*. Blackwell, Oxford.

Swinscow TDV (1998) *Statistics at Square One* (9e). BMJ Publishing Group, London.

Other

O'Connell S (1998) *NANP Handbook for Non-Principals*. Limited Edition Press. London.

Useful addresses

British Medical Association
Tavistock Square
London WC1H 9JP
(020) 7387 4499
Web: http://www.bma.org.uk

General Medical Council
44 Hallam Street
London W1N 6EA
(020) 7580 7642

Royal College of General Practitioners
14 Princes Gate
London SW7 1PU
(020) 7581 3232
Web: http://www.rcgp.org.uk

Joint Committee for Postgraduate Training in General Practice
14 Princes Gate
London SW7 1PU
(020) 7581 3232

National Association of Non-Principals
PO Box 188
Chichester
West Sussex
PO19 2ZA
Email: info@nanp.org.uk
Web: http://www.nanp.org.uk

Index